SirtFood

DIET

Change Your Eating Habits, Activate Your Skinny Gene and Burn Fat! A Complete Beginner's Guide with Quick and Easy Delicious Recipes for Rapid Weight Loss.

Andrew William

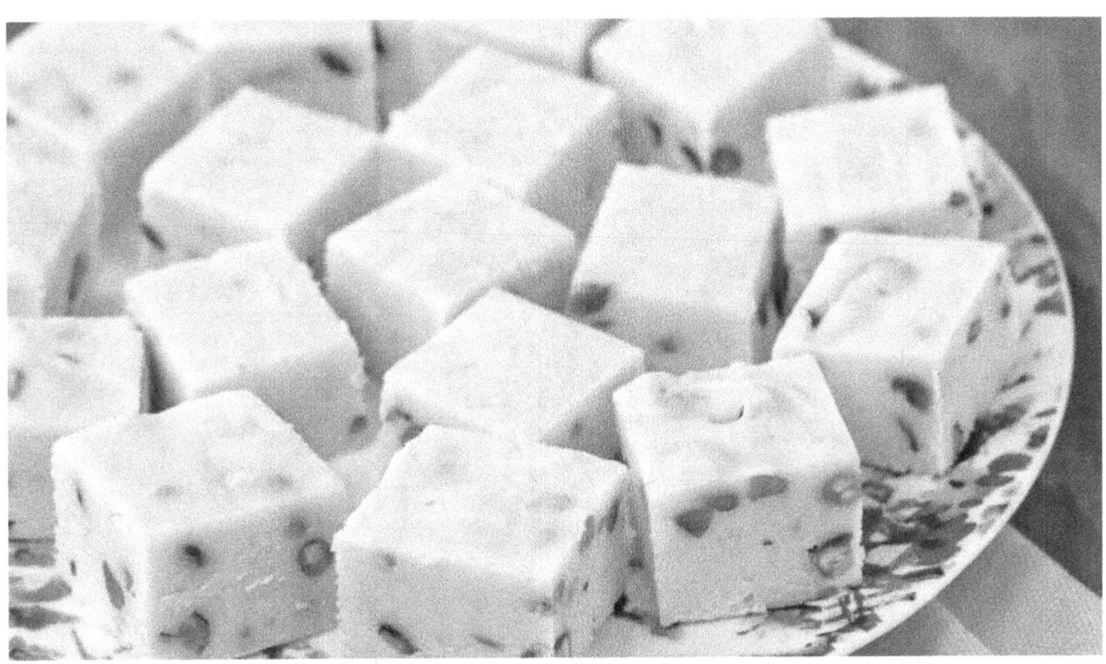

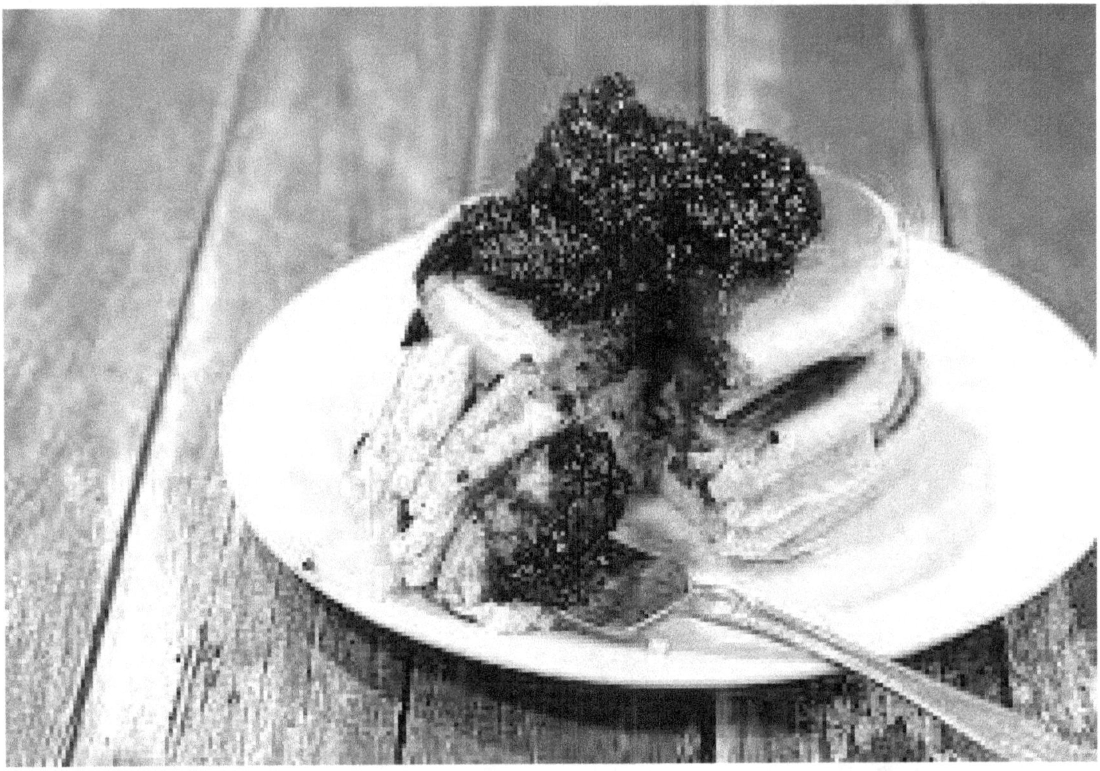

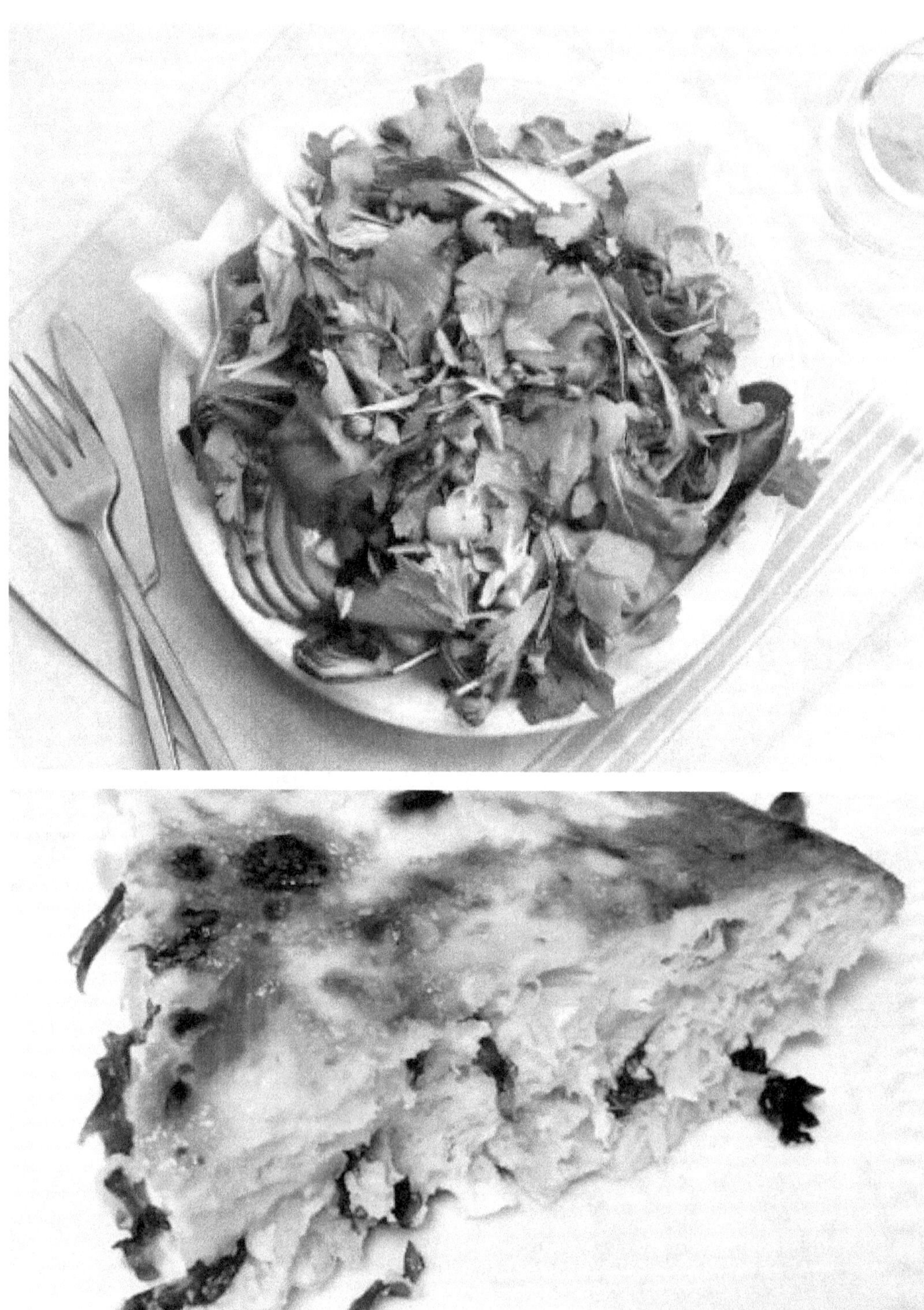

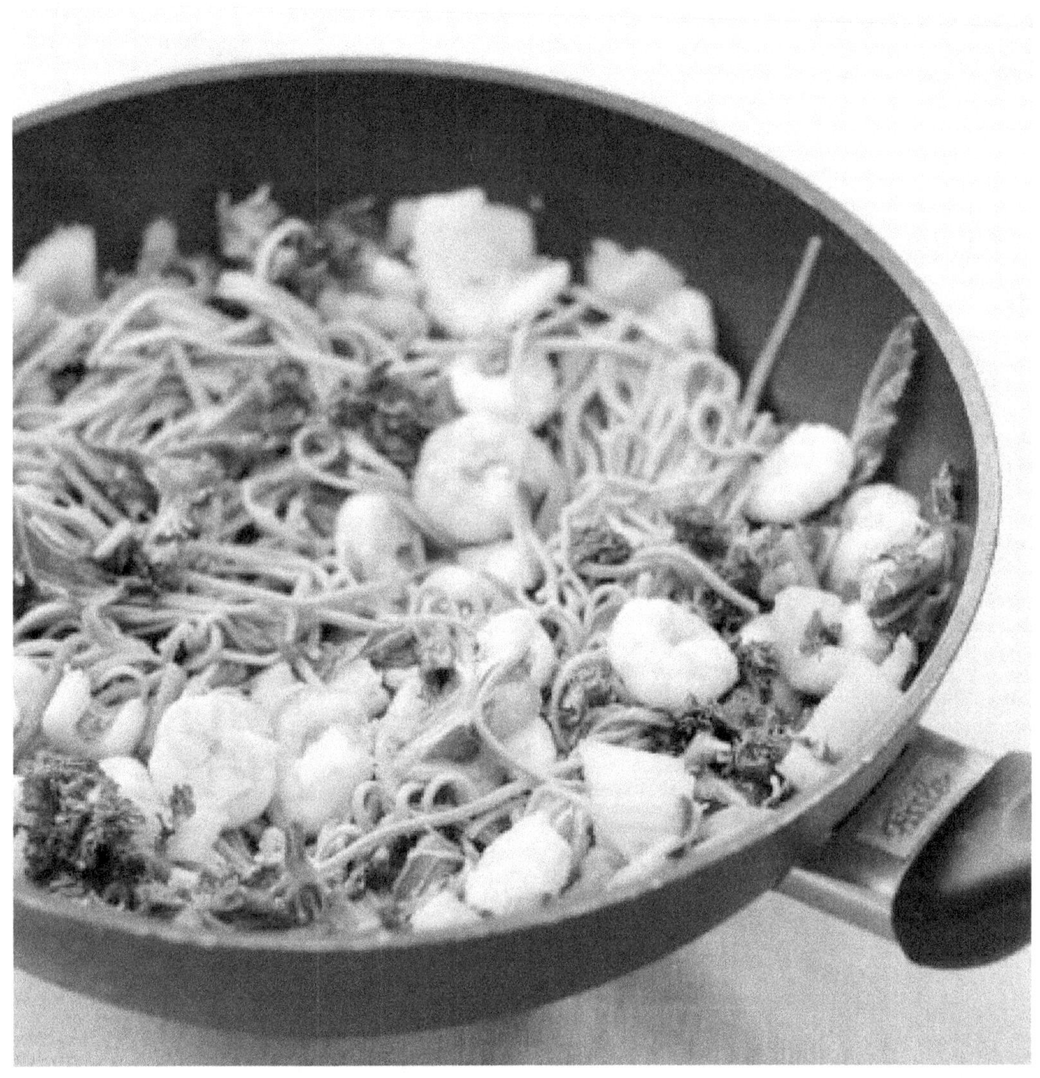

CONTENTS

Introduction 1

   Fun Facts about Sirtuins: 2

   To Sum Up 2

   Is This the Diet for You? 3

   The Discovery and History of Sirtuins . 3

What is Sirtfood Diet 1

   What Is the Master Strategy? 1

   What Does This Promise? 1

   Does this convey? 1

   What Would You Be Able to spend? 1

   What Should You Avoid Consuming? .. 2

   Sirtfood Diet Claims 3

   Evidence of Your Sirtfood Diet 3

   Tiny sample-size 4

   Sample bias 4

   No follow-up 4

   No control groups 5

   Calories restriction 5

   The Verdict on The Sirtfood Diet 5

Lifestyle Advice 7

   Lifestyle Advice 7

   Meal Plan 9

     Phase 1 Meal Plan 9

     Phase 2 Meal Plan 10

Phase 1 Breakfast Recipes 11

   1.   Chocolate Granola 11

   2.   Chocolate Waffles 12

   3.   Salmon & Kale Omelet 13

   4.   Kale Scramble 14

   5.   Eggs with Kale 15

   6.   Green Omelet 16

   7.   Smoked Salmon Omelet 17

   8.   Pancakes with Apples and Blackcurrants 18

   9.   Granola 19

   10.   Pistachio fudge 20

Phase 1 Lunch Recipes 21

   11.   Butternut Pumpkin with Buckwheat 21

   12.   Chicken and Kale with Spicy Salsa 22

   13.   Cucumber & Onion Salad 23

   14.   Citrus Fruit Salad 24

   15.   Mixed Berries Salad 25

   16.   Orange & Beet Salad 26

   17.   Strawberry, Apple & Arugula Salad 27

   18.   Shrimp Salad 28

19. Smoked Salmon Sirt Salad 29

20. Tofu & Shiitake Mushroom Soup 30

21. Kale & Shiitake Stew 31

22. Kale & Chicken Stew.................32

Phase 1 Snack Recipe 33

23. Fruity Granola Bars 33

24. Cardamom Granola Bars 34

25. Coconut Brownie Bites 35

26. Tortilla Chips and Fresh Salsa..36

27. Garlic Baked Kale Chips...........37

28. Herb Roasted Chickpeas...........38

29. Cauliflower Nachos...................39

Phase 1 Dinner Recipes 41

30. Kale White Bean Pork Soup.....41

31. Turkey Satay Skewers 42

32. Salmon & Capers.......................43

33. Moroccan Chicken Casserole ...44

34. Vegetable broth 45

35. Chicken Broth............................46

36. Beef Broth.................................47

37. Chili Con Carne 49

38. Prawn & Coconut Curry 50

39. Chicken & Bean Casserole........51

40. Sesame Miso Chicken................52

Phase 2 Breakfast Recipes 54

41. Salmon Sirt Super Salad 54

42. Sirtfood Granola 55

43. Red Onion Dhal.........................56

44. Tomato Frittata 57

45. Choc Chip Granola....................58

46. Horseradish Flaked Salmon Fillet & Kale..59

47. Apple Pancakes with Blackcurrant Compote 60

48. Strawberry Buckwheat Tabbouleh 61

49. Buckwheat Pasta Salad..............62

Phase 2 Lunch Recipes 63

50. Tuscan Bean Stew......................63

51. Chinese-Style Pork with Pak Choi 64

52. . Lamb, Butternut Squash and Date Tagine..65

53. Chargrilled Beef with A Red Wine Jus, Onion Rings, Garlic Kale, and Herb Simmered Potatoes......................66

54. Turmeric Baked Salmon 68

55. Prawn & Chili Pak Choi 69

Phase 2 Snacks 71

56. Tuna Salad 71

57. Kale & Feta Salad 72

58. Buckwheat Pasta Salad 73

59. Sesame Chicken Salad 74

60. Sirt Fruit Salad 75

61. Crowning Celebration Chicken Salad 76

62. Sirt Super Salad 77

Phase 2 Dinner Recipes 79

63. Asian king prawn stir-fry with buckwheat noodles 79

64. Greek Salad Skewers 80

65. Sirtfood Cauliflower Couscous & Turkey Steak 81

66. Miso Caramelized Tofu 82

67. King Prawn Stir-fry & Soba 83

68. Mushroom & Tofu Scramble ... 84

69. Fragrant Asian Hotpot 85

70. Greek salad skewers 86

71. Sweet-smelling Chicken Breast with Kale, Red Onion, and Salsa 87

72. Tuscan Bean Stew 88

Bonus Phase 2 Recipes 89

73. Sirtfood bites 89

74. Sirt Muesli 90

75. Raspberry and Blackcurrant Jelly 91

76. Sirtfood Mushroom Scramble Eggs 92

77. Sirtfood Scrambled Eggs 93

78. Fragrant Asian Hotpot 94

79. Turkey With Cauliflower Cous 95

10 Juices and Smoothies 97

80. Sirtfood Cocktail 97

81. Summer Berry Smoothie 98

82. Mango, Celery & Ginger Smoothie 99

83. Orange, Carrot & Kale Smoothie 100

84. Creamy Strawberry & Cherry Smoothie 101

85. Grape, Celery & Parsley Reviver 102

86. Strawberry & Citrus Blend 103

87. Grapefruit & Celery Blast 104

88.   Orange & Celery Crush...........105

89.   Tropical Chocolate Delight 106

Bonus Recipes 107

90.   Buckwheat Porridge.................107

91.   Chocolate Granola 108

92.   Blueberry Muffins 109

93.   Chocolate Waffles 110

94.   Salmon & Kale Omelet...........111

95.   Eggs with Kale.........................112

Exercising....................................113

Combining Exercise with the Sirtfood Diet.....................................113

The SirtDiet Principles 113

Exercise During The First Few Weeks 113

When The Diet Becomes A Lifestyle 113

Home body weight circuit training:...114

After Diet...................................117

Conclusion 123

Introduction

The sirtfood diet can't be classified as low-carb or low-fat. This diet differs greatly from its many precursors while advocating many of the same things: the ingestion of fresh plant-based foods. As the name implies, this is a sirtuin based diet, but what are sirtuins, and why have you never heard about them before?

There are seven sirtuin proteins – SIRT-1 to SIRT-71. They can be found throughout your cells and the cells of every animal on the planet. Sirtuins are found in almost every living organism and in almost every part of the cell, controlling what goes on. Supplement company, Elysium Health, likens the body's cells to an office with sirtuins acting as the CEO, helping the cells react to internal and external changes. They govern what is done when it's done, and who does is.

Of the seven sirtuins, one works in your cell's cytoplasm, three in the cell's mitochondria, and another three in the cell's nucleus. They have a wide number of jobs to perform, but mostly they remove acetyl groups from other proteins. These acetyl groups signal that the protein they are attached to is available to perform its function. Sirtuins remove the flag and get the protein ready to use.

Sirtuins sound crucial to your body's normal function, so why is that you've never heard of them before?

The first sirtuin to be discovered was SIR2, a gene discovered in the 1970s which controlled the ability of fruit flies to mate. It wasn't until the 1990s that scientists discovered other similar proteins in almost every form of life. Every organism had a different number of sirtuins – bacteria has one, and yeast has five. Experiments on mice show they have the same number as humans, seven.

Sirtuins have been shown to prolong life in yeast and in mice. There is, so far, no evidence of the same effect in human beings; however, these sirtuins are present in almost every form of life, and many scientists hope that if organisms as far apart as yeast and mice can see the same effect from sirtuin activation, this may also extend to humans.

Besides sirtuins, our bodies need another substance called nicotinamide adenine dinucleotide for cells to function properly. Elysium (see above) likens this substance to the money a company needs to keep operating. Like any CEO, a sirtuin can only keep the company working properly if the cash flow is sufficient. NAD+ was first discovered in 1906. You get your supply of NAD+ from your diet by eating foods made up the building blocks of NAD+.

Fun Facts about Sirtuins:

1. Mice that have been engineered to have top levels of SIRT-1 are both more active and leaner than normal, while mice that lack SIRT-1 altogether are fatter and more prone to various metabolic conditions.
2. Add the fact that levels of SIRT-1 are much lower in obese people than in those of a "healthy" weight, and the case for the importance of sirtuins in weight loss becomes interesting.
3. By changing your diet and adding the best sirtfoods to your eating plan, the authors of the sirtfood diet believe everyone can achieve better health, all without losing muscle mass.

To Sum Up

Exercise and calories restriction are both sources of stress which encourage our bodies to adapt to changing circumstances. If the stress becomes too great, the result can be an injury, the body can even die, but at lower levels, we adapt, and this temporary, low-level stress is key to many physiological changes. For example, stress on muscles, enough but not too much, is what makes the body increase muscle mass.

Similarly, the authors of the sirtfood diet found that it is when the body is stressed, by exercise or low-calories intake, that the effect of sirtuins kicks in, and it is this effect that can be reproduced by a diet rich in SIRT foods.

Any diet plan you adopt involves some level of expense and inconvenience. It may also involve risk. Anyone can write a diet book, as there is no need to have the diet medically approved. That's one reason all diets start by suggesting you consult a doctor. One thing you can do is look at the qualifications of the diet's author.

The authors of the sirtfood diet are not TV personalities or reality stars. They have genuine scientific knowledge of the subject, and both have Master's degrees to prove it.

Aidan Goggins is a pharmacist with a degree in pharmacy and a Master's degree in Nutritional Medicine. Glen Matten trained at the Institute for Optimum Nutrition before completing his Master's degree in nutritional medicine.

The sirtfood diet is not their first collaboration. In 2012, they wrote, "The Health Delusion," a book that attacked many of the "long-held truths" of the diet and health industry. As a result, they received the consumer health book of the year award by the Medical Journalists Association.

Having reviewed the literature and asked the enormous question: "What would happen if we ate sirtfoods? Would there be weight loss?" they asked: "What would happen to muscle mass, which is usually lost during almost any diet?"

To find the answers, the authors conducted a trial in an exclusive health spa near London in the UK. There were 40 participants. 39 completed the trial. Because the trial was carried out at a health spa, the authors had complete control over the food eaten by the participants. Note that this is not always the case in "medical" trials where the participants report what they ate.

The Discovery and History of Sirtuins

There were different quantities of sirtuins in every creature. For instance, yeast has five sirtuins, microscopic organisms have one, mice have seven, and people have seven.

How sirtuins were found across species implies they were "saved" with development. Qualities that are "rationed" have all-inclusive capacities in many or all species. What was at this point to be known, however, was the means by which significant sirtuins would end up being.

In 1991, Elysium fellow benefactor and MIT scholar Leonard Guarente, nearby alumni understudies Nick Austriaco and Brian Kennedy, led trials to even more likely see how yeast matured. By some coincidence, Austriaco attempted to develop societies of different yeast strains from tests he had put away in his ice chest for quite a long time, which made a distressing domain for the strains. Just a portion of these strains could develop from here, yet Guarente and his group identified an example: The strains of yeast that endure the best in the cooler were likewise the longest-lived. This gave direction to Guarente so he could concentrate only on these long-living strains of yeast.

This prompted the identification of SIR2 as a quality that advanced life span in yeast. It's critical to note more research is required on SIR2's belongings in people. The Guarantee lab consequently found that expelling SIR2 abbreviated yeast life range significantly, while in particular, expanding the number of duplicates of the SIR2 quality from one to two expanded the life length in yeast. What started SIR2 normally presently couldn't seem to be found.

This is the place acetyl bunches become possibly the most important factor. It was at first idea that SIR2 might be a deacetylating protein — which means it expelled those acetyl gatherings — from different atoms, yet nobody knew if this were valid since all endeavors to show this movement in a test tube demonstrated negative. Guarantee and his group had the option to find that SIR2 in yeast could just deacetylate different proteins within sight of the coenzyme NAD+, nicotinamide adenine dinucleotide.

In Guarente's own words: "Without NAD+, SIR2 sits idle. That was the basic finding on the circular segment of sirtuin science."

What is Sirtfood Diet

What Is the Master Strategy?

There are 2 stages for the sirtfood day by day diet. The principal goes on for a week, the following for 14 days. Throughout the initial three days of this all-inclusive strategy, you are restricted to 1000 calories out of one feast of sirtfoods alongside likewise 3 green juices. For the rest of the primary week, at that point, you additionally can gobble up 2 green squeezes alongside 2 sirtfood suppers consistently. During the stage, the eating regimen plan comprises three sirtfood suppers besides likewise 1 green juice.

What Does This Promise?

On the off chance that you truly don't cheapen the end-all strategy, the sirtfood diet keeps up a seven-pound bodyweight reduction from the underlying week (without relinquishing muscles). Also, it professes to decrease hostile to maturing impacts, to help improve memory and blood glucose control and lower the chance of incessant disease.

Does this convey?

The exploration of the capacity of a sirtuin is truly restricted - most of the lab concentrate between yeast, lab creatures, and undeveloped human cells. Polyphenol ingestion has precisely the same great impact on the human metabolic rate because of calories constraint. Before this dietary system is really breaking down in human clinical preliminaries, at that point, it's impractical to state with any assurance of how individuals could toll.

What Would You Be Able to spend?

Although some sirtfoods are ordinary in practically pretty much any general store or well-being food store (and could be in your kitchen), the others might not be easy to find.

"Sirtfoods incorporates kale, dim chocolate, red wine, cherry powder, onions, garlic, parsley, pecans, garlic, and berries. A considerable lot of these fixings are easy to get and, in this way, are notable as solid decisions. Extra fixings could be harder to source, for example, lovage, buckwheat, and matcha green tea **extricate** powder."

Officially, no foods have been "barred" on the sirtfood diet; however, the calories limitation remains serious —mainly during the first three days when you are restricted by 1000 calories.

The toughest portion of this sirtfood diet is calories limitation and the dependence on green juice, and also, this has the potential to be dangerous for several forms of individuals possibly. It's not suggested for people on several medications, such as Coumadin, or even with medical conditions such as diabetes. It should also be avoided by those who are nursing or pregnant.

Sirtuins are a class of proteins present in living entities – including humans – which research has proved to take part in essential biological processes like aging, cellular death, inflammation, and metabolism.

On the flip side, sirtuins may live longer, and in line with their own proponents, they could also allow you to lose body fat. The expectation is that eating a slew of sirtfoods will trigger the sirtuin genes (sometimes called lean genes) similar to flaxseed.

However, does this work like that? Some background: "in mammals, there are seven kinds of sirtuins, that vary between sirt1 and sirt7. Of these, sirt1 will be the one which researchers are interested in," states Sims. "Sirt1 is occasionally called the protector against oxidative stress and DNA damage."

This sirtfood diet is whether you're able to trigger sirt1, you're able to produce more mitochondria, the powerhouse of these cells, that may decrease oxidative stress, letting you age quicker.

The problem? "You cannot possibly eat up enough of these foods recommended by this daily diet plan to increase sirtuins. For example, red wine, which will be within this sirtfood diet: to receive 20 mg of resveratrol [an antioxidant that arouses sirt1], you must drink much over 40 glasses of wine." We are not suggesting you do that.

Can it be said that the sirtfood diet is a sure secret to fat reduction in the very long haul? We examine the research supporting the popular sirtfood diet with others and research on whether it works for weight loss.

The biggest claim that the dietary plan boasts concerning is these sirtuin proteins increase the body's capacity to burn off fat and boost muscle development, maintenance, and repair so that as cited earlier – sped up weight reduction. As sped up, fat reduction is almost always safe, ideal?! (Insert gigantic eye roster). Additional non-weight relevant benefits comprise improving memory, controlling glucose levels, and protecting you from cancer and chronic diseases.

Thus, what's the skinny on these slender genes?

Can it be the sirtfood diet that the secret to fat reduction in the very long haul? We examined the research supporting the popular sirtfood diet and other diets, and research on whether it works for weight loss.

The vast majority of studies studying the aftereffects of sirtuins and fat reduction have just been achieved on endometriosis, viruses, yeast, and individual stem cells. Some yeast and mice studies also have revealed an antioxidant called resveratrol, found in berries and polyphenols that trigger sirtuins, which then can mimic the activities of caloric restriction, which consequently will reduce fat. Original studies have discovered that resveratrol can play a part in cancer prevention, cardiovascular problems, and diabetes in animals. But there is insufficient evidence to comprehend its own function in humans. Still, another thing to explain is that lots of the studies used are examining the isolated form of sirtuins and perhaps not sirtuins seen from the foodstuff, which separates us more from accurately analyzing results. In addition, they often make use of high doses of antioxidants impossible for people to achieve out of food sources (more wine will not equal greater benefits... inclined to be the bearer of terrible news).

The sole human signs round the potency of sirt food diet weight loss originate in a clinical trial. This trial has been comprised of the sirtfood diet publication and created by the creators. Sadly, the clinical trial performed poorly in many areas. The pilot study was 40 participants at a private fitness center in Chelsea, London. Within a seven-day time period, 3-9 participants lost seven lbs, and also their muscle tissue was maintained or increased.

Tiny sample-size

Pilot studies are renowned for being small, thus the definition of pilot analysis, but we can't confidently suggest this dietary plan depending on the impact it had on 39 gym-participants. A pilot study would be the very first of numerous studies that ought to be run to some particular topic, and if on no account, be the sole real source of evidence in making the scenario for a diet regime.

Sample bias

The only participants from the analysis were hard heart health goers who're likely a health-conscious people who follow a nutritious eating plan and exercise regularly. Obviously, its populace is an unbiased representation of the remainder of humankind and is far from reality.

No follow-up

A key dimension to check the efficacy of an appraisal is to look for a follow-up. Like that, it's possible to examine all the participants and also determine if there aren't any long-term benefits. As an alternative, they simply quantified the participants for a week, and then that was it. It will not reveal whether the diet is proven to work.

I have a great deal of beef for this specific restriction. The gist of a clinical trial will be a controller set. Without one, you can't state for sure if the intervention, even in this event, the sirtfood activators, had an immediate effect on the analysis outcomes. Sounds just like whole academic anarchy!

All of these constraints result in quite a feeble study, plus it is apparently the sole study these creators are clinging to. Therefore, that is a huge red flag.

Here is my problem with this specific diet program. Besides resveratrol, something else which can activate sirtuins is restricting calories that explain the reason why it's a part of Phase 1 of this diet program.

Calories restriction

Time and time, I have stated for you guys the exact issue with most diet plans: prohibitive ingestion. If it has to do with limitation, our rebel instincts wish to cheat and binge like mad. I am convinced you can also become that friend that nobody would like to head out with for the "hangry" personality. However, also for understanding, there have yet to be enough consistent studies that state calories limitation could be your thing to do. It's true that you are going to eliminate some candy poundage temporarily. However, additionally, you will meet some unwelcome consequences and finally regain the fat lost. Studies appearing at metabolic restriction discovered that as time passes, limitation contributes to lack in muscular tissue (which completely raises exactly what the sirtfood diet maintains that it could perform), muscular strength and decrease in bone, nausea, vomiting, and depression.

The Verdict on The Sirtfood Diet

In case you prefer sirtfood activators, go right ahead and absorb them. I don't have any problem with boosting an assortment of wholesome foods full of health-protecting angels. I really like a glass of wine by the conclusion of a busy week and that I will not say no to a slice of chocolate. A fantastic guideline is not to anticipate diet plans which converse about losing seven pounds in seven days. To start with, it's generally biased and false advertisements, and second, the vast majority of the full time that it's unsafe. Unlike Adele, the majority folks have no access to elaborate coaches and/or enough full time to get two-a-day fitness center sessions. For the time being, we could say that the research doesn't prefer using sirtuins for weight reduction. For the time being, at least.

Lifestyle Advice

The Sirtfood diet was an achievement nourishment system a couple of years and was the dear eating routine with the broadsheet press at the time. In the event that you missed it, the features are that it incorporates red wine, chocolate, and espresso. Far less promoted and eye-catching (yet similarly uplifting news as we would like to think) is the way that the response to the inquiry, 'would you be able to eat meat on the sirt nourishment diet?', is a resonating, yes.

The eating routine arrangement not just incorporates a decent sound part of the meat; it proceeds to recommend that protein is a basic consideration in a Sirtfood-based eating routine to receive the greatest reward.

We're not supporting this as some meat overwhelming eating routine (we despite everything recollect the awful breath from Atkins), it's in reality very veggie-lover cordial and provides food for practically everybody, which is the thing that makes it so reasonable an alternative to us.

So, what is the Sirtfood diet? It was created by nutritionists Aidan Goggins and Glen Matten, following a pilot learn at the elite XK Gym (Daniel Craig, Madonna, and an entire host of different celebs are supposedly individuals) where they are the two experts in Sloane Square, London. Members in the preliminary lost 7lbs in the initial seven days, in what the creators call the hyper-achievement to organize. The science behind Sirtfoods drops out of an investigation in 2003 which found that a compound found in red wine, expanded the life expectancy of yeast. At last, this prompted the investigations which clarify the medical advantages of red wine, and how (whenever drank reasonably) individuals who drink red wine put on less weight.

A significant part of the science behind the Sirtfood diet is like that of 'fasting-diets' which have been well known for as far back as barely any years, whereby our bodies initiate qualities and our fat stockpiling is turned off; our bodies basically change to endurance mode, thus weight reduction. The negatives to fasting-eats fewer carbs are the unavoidable craving that results, alongside a decrease in vitality, bad-tempered conduct (when you're "hangry"), weariness, and muscle misfortune. The Sirtfood diet professes to counter those negatives, as it's anything but a quick, so hunger isn't an issue, making it ideal for individuals who need to lead a functioning solid way of life.

Sirtfoods are a (generally newfound) gathering of nourishments that are incredible in actuating the 'sirtuin' qualities in our body, which are the qualities enacted in fasting eats fewer carbs. Leucine is an amino corrosive found in protein, which praises and really upgrades the activities of Sirtfoods. This implies the ideal approach to eat Sirtfoods is by consolidating them with a chicken bosom, steak, or another wellspring of leucine, for example, fish or eggs.

Generally, we can thoroughly observe the advantage and intrigue of the Sirtfood diet. Like practically any eating regimen plan, it tends to be a faff getting every one of the fixings, and the 'Sirtfood green juice,' which shapes a centerpiece of the initial 14 days of the arrangement, is a torment to make and really costly, yet it shows improvement over you'd anticipate. We just trialed a couple of days of the arrangement, and keeping in mind that there was perceptible weight reduction, the genuine advantage of the book is the reasonable Direction of bringing Sirtfoods into your regular dinner arranging.

Phase 1 Meal Plan

	Breakfast	Lunch	Dinner
Day 1	Matcha Green Juice	Kale Soup	Buckwheat Noodles with Veggies
Day 2	Kale Scramble	Strawberry, Apple & Arugula Salad	Prawns with Asparagus
Day 3	Blueberry Muffins	Orange & Beet Salad	Kale with tofu & Chickpeas
Day 4	Kale & Orange Smoothie	Sautéed Mushrooms	Shrimp with Kale
Day 5	Chocolate Waffles	Kale Soup	Buckwheat Noodles with Veggies
Day 6	Buckwheat Pancakes	Kale with Pine Nuts	Mushroom & Bok Choy Stir Fry
Day 7	Lemony Apple Juice	Buckwheat Burgers	Shrimp Salad

Phase 2 Meal Plan

	Breakfast	Lunch	Dinner
Day 1	Apple, Orange & Broccoli Juice	Salmon Burgers	Lentils & Greens Soup
Day 2	Mushroom & Kale Frittata	Chickpeas with Swiss Chard	Chicken with Veggies
Day 3	Buckwheat Granola	Arugula, Strawberry & Orange Salad	Lamb Chops with Kale
Day 4	Strawberry Smoothie	Tofu & Broccoli Curry	Chicken & Berries Salad
Day 5	Tofu, Kale & Mushroom Muffins	Salmon Burgers	Chicken & Veggies with Buckwheat Noodles
Day 6	Matcha Pancakes	Arugula, Strawberry & Orange Salad	Steak with Veggies
Day 7	Apple, Grape & Carrot Juice	Chickpeas with Swiss Chard	Shrimp with Veggies

Phase 1 Breakfast Recipes

1. Chocolate Granola

Preparation Time: 10 minutes

Cooking Time: 38 minutes

Servings: 8

Ingredients:

¼ cup cacao powder

¼ cup maple syrup

2 tablespoons coconut oil, melted

½ teaspoon vanilla extract

1/8 teaspoon salt

2 cups gluten-free rolled oats

¼ cup unsweetened coconut flakes

2 tablespoons chia seeds

2 tablespoons unsweetened dark chocolate, chopped finely

Nutrition:

Calories 193

Total Fat 9.1 g

Saturated Fat 5.2 g

Cholesterol 0 mg

Sodium 37 mg

Total Carbs 26.1 g

Fiber 4.6 g

Sugar 5.9 g

Protein 5 g

Directions:

Preheat your oven to 300°F. Line a medium baking sheet with parchment paper. In a medium pan, add the cacao powder, maple syrup, coconut oil, vanilla extract, and salt and mix well. Now, place the pan over medium heat and cook for about 2-3 minutes or until thick and syrupy, stirring continuously. Remove the pan of the mixture from the heat and set aside. In a large bowl, add the oats, coconut, and chia seeds and mix well. Add the syrup mixture and mix until well combined. Transfer the granola mixture onto a prepared baking sheet and spread in an even layer. Bake for approximately 35 minutes. Remove the baking sheet from the oven and set aside for about 1 hour. Add the chocolate pieces and stir to combine. Serve immediately.

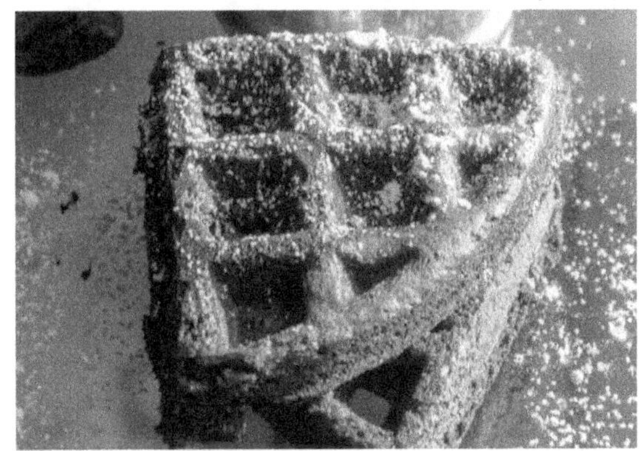

2. Chocolate Waffles

Preparation Time: 15 minutes

Cooking Time: 24 minutes

Servings: 8

Ingredients:

2 cups unsweetened almond milk

1 tablespoon fresh lemon juice

1 cup buckwheat flour

½ cup cacao powder

¼ cup flaxseed meal

1 teaspoon baking soda

1 teaspoon baking powder

¼ teaspoons kosher salt

2 large eggs

½ cup coconut oil, melted

¼ cup dark brown sugar

2 teaspoons vanilla extract

2 ounces unsweetened dark chocolate, chopped roughly

Nutrition:

Calories 295

Total Fat 22.1 g

Saturated Fat 15.5 g

Cholesterol 47 mg

Sodium 302 mg

Total Carbs 1.5 g

Fiber 5.2 g

Sugar 5.1 g

Protein 6.3 g

Direction:

In a bowl, add the almond milk and lemon juice and mix well. Set aside for about 10 minutes. In a bowl, place buckwheat flour, cacao powder, flaxseed meal, baking soda, baking powder, and salt and mix well. In the bowl of the almond milk mixture, place the eggs, coconut oil, brown sugar, and vanilla extract and beat until smooth. Now, place the flour mixture and beat until smooth. Gently fold in the chocolate pieces. Preheat the waffle iron and then grease it. Place the desired amount of the mixture into the preheated waffle iron and cook for about 3 minutes or until golden brown. Repeat with the remaining mixture. Serve warm.

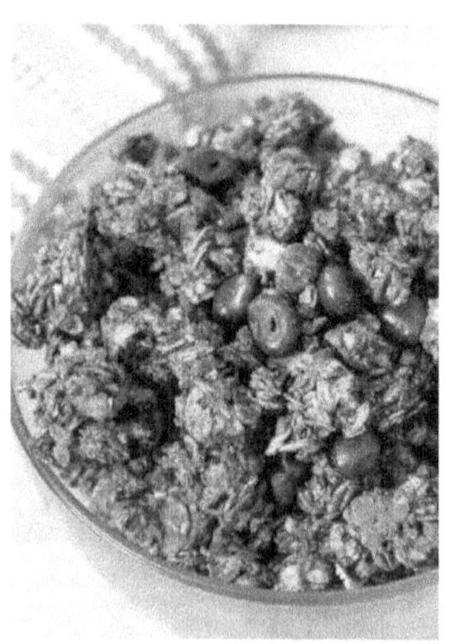

Preparation Time: 10 minutes

Cooking Time: 7 minutes

Servings: 4

Ingredients:

6 eggs

2 tablespoons unsweetened almond milk

Salt and ground black pepper, as required

2 tablespoons olive oil

4 ounces smoked salmon, cut into bite-sized chunks

2 cup fresh kale, tough ribs removed and chopped finely

4 scallions, chopped finely

Directions:

In a bowl, place the eggs, coconut milk, salt, and black pepper and beat well. Set aside. In a nonstick wok, heat the oil over medium heat. Place the egg mixture evenly and cook for about 30 seconds without stirring. Place the salmon kale and scallions on top of the egg mixture evenly. Now, adjust the heat to low and cook, covered for about 4-5 minutes or until omelet is done completely. Uncover the wok and cook for about 1 minute. Carefully transfer the omelet onto a serving plate and serve.

Nutrition:

Calories 210

Total Fat 14.9 g

Saturated Fat 3.3 g

Cholesterol 252 mg

Sodium 682 mg

Total Carbs 5.2 g

Fiber 0.9 g

Sugar 0.9 g

Protein 14.8 g

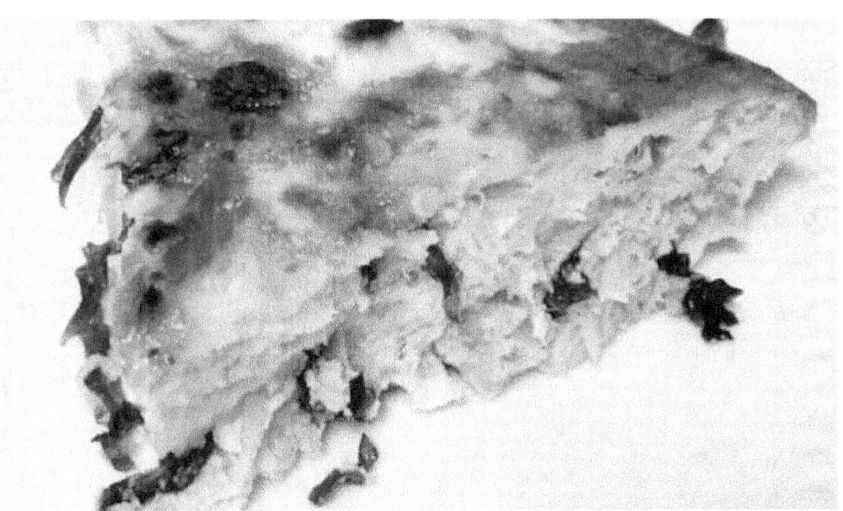

4. Kale Scramble

Preparation Time: 10 minutes

Cooking Time: 6 minutes

Servings: 2

Ingredients:

4 eggs

1/8 teaspoon ground turmeric

Salt and ground black pepper, as required

1 tablespoon water

2 teaspoons olive oil

1 cup fresh kale, tough ribs removed and chopped

Directions:

In a bowl, place eggs, turmeric, salt, black pepper, and water and with a whisk, beat until foamy. In a wok, heat the oil over medium heat. Stir in the egg mixture and immediately reduce the heat to medium-low. Cook for about 1-2 minutes, stirring frequently. Stir in the kale and cook for about 3-4 minutes, stirring frequently. Remove the wok from heat and serve immediately.

Nutrition:

Calories 183

Total Fat 13.4 g

Saturated Fat 3.4 g

Cholesterol 327 mg

Sodium 216 mg

Total Carbs 4.3 g

Fiber 0.5 g

Sugar 0.7 g

Protein 12.1 g

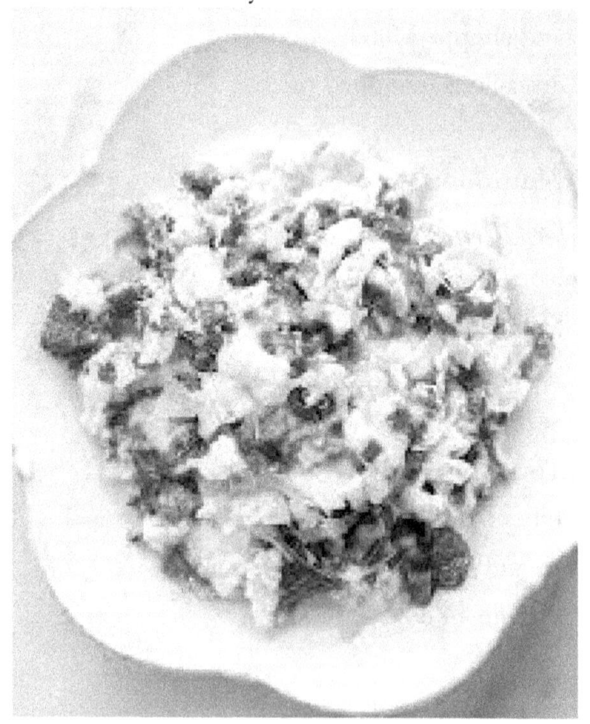

Preparation Time: 15 minutes

Cooking Time: 25 minutes

Servings: 4

Ingredients:

2 tablespoons olive oil

1 red onion, chopped

2 garlic cloves, minced

1 cup tomatoes, chopped

½ pound fresh kale, tough ribs removed and chopped

1 teaspoon ground cumin

¼ teaspoon red pepper flakes, crushed

Salt and ground black pepper, as required

4 eggs

2 tablespoons fresh parsley, chopped

Directions: Heat the oil in a large wok over medium heat and sauté the onion for about 4-5 minutes. Add garlic and sauté for about 1 minute. Add the tomatoes, spices, salt and black pepper and cook for about 2-3 minutes, stirring frequently. Stir in the kale and cook for about 4-5 minutes. Carefully, crack eggs on top of the kale mixture. With the lid, cover the wok and cook for about 10 minutes or until the desired doneness of eggs. Serve hot with the garnishing of parsley.

Nutrition:

Calories 175

Total Fat 11.7 g

Saturated Fat 2.4 g

Cholesterol 164 mg

Sodium 130 mg

Total Carbs 11.5 g

Fiber 2.2 g

Sugar 2.8 g

Protein 8.2 g

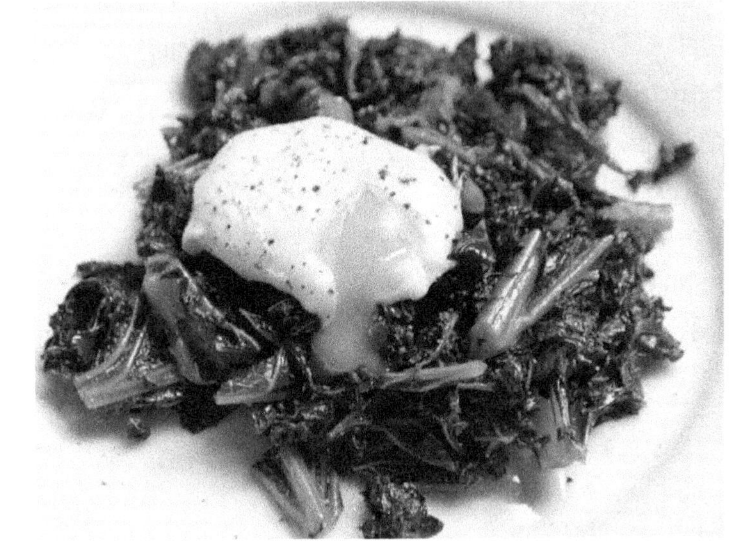

Preparation Time: 10 min

Cooking Time: 5 min

Servings: 1

Ingredients:

2 large eggs, at room temperature

1 shallot, peeled and chopped

Handful arugula

3 sprigs of parsley, chopped

1 tsp extra virgin olive oil

Salt and black pepper

Directions:

Beat the eggs in a small bowl and set aside. Sauté the shallot for 5 minutes with a bit of the oil on low-medium heat. Pour the eggs in the pans, stirring the mixture for just a second. The eggs on medium heat, and tip the pan just enough to let the loose egg run underneath after about one minute on the burner. Add the greens, herbs, and the seasonings to the top side as it is still soft. TIP: You do not even have to flip it, as you can just cook the egg slowly egg as is well.

TIP: Another option is to put it into an oven to broil for 3-5 minutes (checking to make sure it is golden but not burned).

Nutrition:

Calories: 234 kcal

Carbs: 25 g

Fat: 72 g

Sodium: 1720 mg

Protein: 64 g

Preparation Time: 5 Minutes

Cooking Time: 45 Minutes

Servings 1

Ingredients

10g of chopped Rocket

100g smoked salmon, sliced

1 teaspoon of extra virgin olive oil

½ teaspoon of capers

2 medium eggs

1 teaspoon of chopped Parsley

Directions

Crack the eggs into a bowl and whisk them well. Add the capers, parsley, rocket, and salmon and heat oil in a non-stick pan until hot but not smoking. Add the egg mixture into the pan and move it around the pan using a spatula. Reduce the heat to low and let the omelet cook. Slide the spatula under the omelet, fold it up in half, and serve.

Nutrition:

Calories: 288.1 kcal

Total Fat: 9.2 g

Cholesterol: 205.6 mg

Sodium: 2,112.5 mg

Potassium: 318.9 mg

Total Carbohydrate: 15.6 g

Dietary Fiber: 3.1 g

Sugars: 0.8 g

Protein: 33.1 g

Preparation Time: 30 min

Cooking Time: 10 min

Servings: 4

Ingredients:

2 apples, cut into small chunks

2 cups of quick-cooking oats

1 cup flour of your choice

1 tsp baking powder

2 tbsp. raw sugar, coconut sugar, or 2 tbsp. honey that is warm and easy to distribute

<u>For the berry topping:</u>

1 cup blackcurrants, washed and stalks removed

3 tbsp. water

2 tbsp. sugar

2 egg whites

1 ¼ cups of milk (or soy/rice/coconut)

2 tsp extra virgin olive oil

A dash of salt

Directions:

Place the ingredients for the topping in a small pot simmer, frequently stirring for about 10 minutes until it cooks down and the juices are released. Take the dry ingredients and mix them in a bowl. After, add the apples and the milk a bit at a time (you may not use it all), until it is a batter. Stiffly whisk the egg whites and then gently mix them into the pancake batter. Set aside in the refrigerator. Pour a one-quarter of the oil onto a flat pan or flat griddle, and when hot, pour some of the batters into it in a pancake shape. When the pancakes start to have golden brown edges and form air bubbles, they may be ready to be gently flipped. Test to be sure the bottom can live away from the pan before actually flipping. Repeat for the next three pancakes. Top each pancake with the berries.

Nutrition:

Calories: 337 kcal

Preparation Time: 30 min

Cooking time: 0 min

Servings: 1

Ingredients:

1 cup buckwheat puffs

1 cup buckwheat flakes (ready to eat type, but not whole buckwheat that needs to be cooked) ½ cup coconut flakes

½ cup Medjool dates, without pits, chopped into smaller, bite-sized pieces

1 cup of cacao nibs or very dark chocolate chips

1/2 cup walnuts, chopped

1 cup strawberries, chopped and without stems 1 cup plain Greek, or coconut or soy yogurt.

Nutrition:

Calories: 140

Fat: 9g

Sodium: 85mg

Carbohydrates: 14g

Fiber: 3g

Sugars: 4g

Protein: 3g

Directions:

Mix, without yogurt and strawberry toppings. You can store it for up to a week. Store in an airtight container. Add toppings (even different berries or different yogurt. You can even use the berry toppings as you will learn how to make from other recipes.

Preparation Time: 10 minutes

Cooking Time: 20 minutes

Servings: 10

Ingredients

225g (8oz) medjool dates

100g (3½ oz) pistachio nuts, shelled (or other nuts)

50g (2oz) desiccated (shredded) coconut

25g (1oz) oats

2 tablespoons water

Nutrition:

Calories: 199.6

Total Fat 10.1 g

Cholesterol 12.5 mg

Sodium 43.4 mg

Total Carbohydrate 26.1 g

Dietary Fiber 0.2 g

Sugars 25.1 g

Protein 2.3 g

Directions

Place the dates, nuts, coconut, oats, and water into a food processor and process until the ingredients are well mixed. Remove the mixture and roll it to 2cm (1 inch) thick. Cut it into 10 pieces and serve.

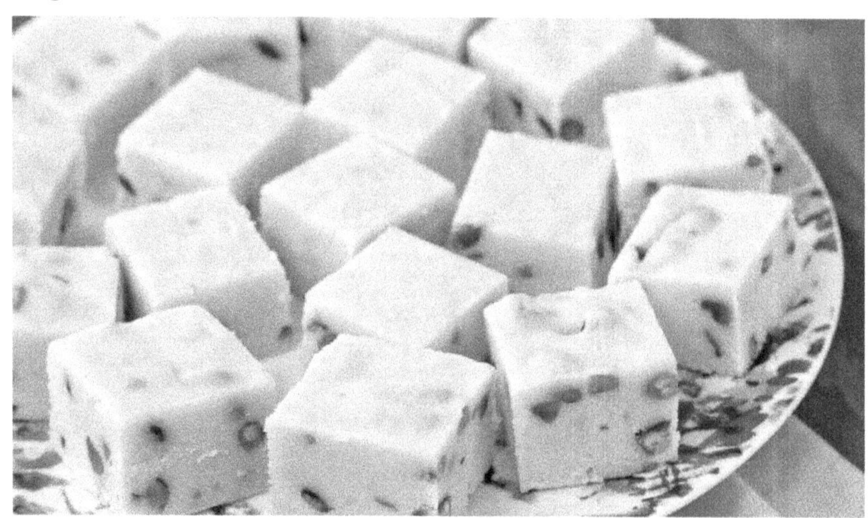

11. Butternut Pumpkin with Buckwheat

Preparation Time: 10 Minutes

Cooking Time: 30 Minutes

Servings: 4

Ingredients

1 tablespoon of extra virgin olive oil

1 red onion, finely chopped

1 tablespoon fresh ginger, finely chopped

3 cloves of garlic, finely chopped

2 small chilies, finely chopped

1 tablespoon cumin

1 cinnamon stick

2 tablespoons turmeric

800g chopped canned tomatoes

300ml vegetable broth

100g dates, seeded and chopped

one 400g tin of chickpeas, drained

500g butter squash, peeled, seeded and cut into pieces

200g buckwheat

5g coriander, chopped

10g parsley, chopped

Directions:

Preheat oven to 400 °. Heat the olive oil in a frying pan and sauté the onion, ginger, garlic, and tai chili. After two minutes, add cumin, cinnamon, and turmeric and cook for another two minutes while stirring. Add the tomatoes, dates, stock, and chickpeas, stir well and cook over low heat for 45 to 60 minutes. Add some water as required. In the meantime, mix the pumpkin pieces with olive oil and bake in the oven for about 30 minutes until soft. Cook the buckwheat according to the Directions and add the remaining turmeric. When everything is cooked, add the pumpkin to the other ingredients in the roaster and serve with the buckwheat. Sprinkle with coriander and parsley.

Nutrition:

Calories: 164 kcal

Carbs: 44 g

Protein: 4 g

Fiber: 14 g

Preparation Time: 10 Minutes

Cooking Time: 50 Minutes

Servings 1

Ingredients:

1 skinless, boneless chicken filet/breast

¼ cup buckwheat

1/4 lemon, juiced

1 tbsp. extra virgin olive oil

1 cup kale, chopped

1/2 red onion, sliced

<u>Salsa:</u>

1 tomato

3 sprigs of parsley, chopped

1 tbsp. chopped capers

1 chili, deseeded and mincedJuice of

1/4 lemon

1 tsp fresh ginger, chopped

2 tsp ground turmeric

Directions:

Chop all ingredients above, just for the salsa, and set aside in a bowl. Pre-eat the oven to 425 F. Add a teaspoon of the turmeric, the lemon juice, and a little oil to the chicken, cover, and set aside for 10 minutes. In a hot pan, slide the chicken and marinade and cook for 2-3 minutes each side, on high to sear it. Then, slide it all onto a baking-safe dish and cook for about 20 minutes or until cooked. Lightly steam the kale in a steamer, or on the stovetop with a lid and some water, for about 5 minutes. You want to wilt the kale, not boil or burn it. Sautee the red onions and ginger, and after 4-5 minutes, add the cooked kale and stir for 1 minute. Cook the buckwheat, adding in the turmeric, see a package or look online if it was bought in bulk. Serve the chicken along with the buckwheat, kale, and spicy salsa.

Nutrition:

Calories 590kcal

Fat 18.6g

Proteins 47.3g

Carbs 57.0g

Preparation Time: 10 minutes

Cooking Time: 0 Minutes

Servings: 4

Ingredients:

3 large cucumbers, sliced thinly

½ cup red onion, sliced

2 tablespoons olive oil

1 tablespoon fresh apple cider vinegar

Sea salt, to taste

¼ cup fresh parsley, chopped

Directions:

In a salad bowl, place all the ingredients and toss to coat well. Serve immediately.

Nutrition:

Calories 81

Total Fat 5.8 g

Saturated Fat 0.9g

Cholesterol 0 mg

Sodium 49 mg

Total Carbs 7.7 g

Fiber 1.2 g

Sugar 3.5 g

Protein 1.3 g

Preparation Time: 15 minutes

Cooking Time: 0 Minutes

Servings: 2

Ingredients:

For Salad:

3 cups fresh kale, tough ribs removed and torn

1 orange, peeled and segmented

1 grapefruit, peeled and segmented

2 tablespoons unsweetened dried cranberries

For Dressing:

2 tablespoons extra-virgin olive oil

2 tablespoons fresh orange juice

1 teaspoon Dijon mustard

½ teaspoon raw honey

Salt and ground black pepper, as required

Directions:

For the salad: in a salad bowl, place all ingredients and mix.

For the dressing: place all ingredients in another bowl and beat until well combined.

Place dressing on top of the salad and toss to coat well. Serve immediately.

Nutrition:

Calories 256

Total Fat 14.5g

Saturated Fat 2.1 g

Cholesterol 0 mg

Sodium 150 mg

Total Carbs 31.3 g

Fiber 4.8 g

Sugar 16.6 g

Protein 4.6 g

Preparations Time: 15 minutes

Cooking Time: 0 Minutes

Servings: 4

Ingredients:

1 cup fresh strawberries, hulled and sliced

½ cup fresh blackberries

½ cup fresh blueberries

½ cup fresh raspberries

6 cups fresh arugula

2 tablespoons extra-virgin olive oil

Salt and ground black pepper, as required

Directions:

In a salad bowl, place all the ingredients and toss to coat well.

Serve immediately.

Nutrition:

Calories 105

Total Fat 7.6 g

Saturated Fat 1 g

Cholesterol 0 mg

Sodium 48 mg

Total Carbs 10.1 g

Fiber 3.6 g

Sugar 5.7 g

Protein 1.6 g

Preparation Time: 15 minutes

Servings: 4

Ingredients:

3 large oranges, peeled, seeded and sectioned

2 beets, trimmed, peeled and sliced

6 cups fresh rocket

¼ cup walnuts, chopped

3 tablespoons olive oil

Pinch of salt

Nutrition:

Calories 233

Total Fat 15.6 g

Saturated Fat 1.8 g

Cholesterol 0 mg

Sodium 86 mg

Total Carbs 23.1 g

Fiber 5.3 g

Sugar 17.6 g

Protein 4.8 g

Directions:

In a salad bowl, place all ingredients and gently, toss to coat.

Serve immediately

Preparation Time: 15 Minutes

Cooking Time: 0 Minutes

Servings: 4

Ingredients:

For Salad:

4 cups fresh baby arugula

2 apples, cored and sliced

1 cup fresh strawberries, hulled and sliced

¼ cup walnuts, chopped

4 tablespoons olive oil

Salt and ground black pepper, as required

Nutrition:

Calories 243

Total Fat 19.1 g

Saturated Fat 2.3 g

Cholesterol 0 mg

Sodium 46 mg

Total Carbs 19.7 g

Fiber 4.3 g

Sugar 13.9 g

Protein 2.9 g

Directions:

For the salad, place all the ingredients in a large bowl and mix well.

For the dressing, place all the ingredients in a bowl and beat until well combined.

Pour the dressing over the salad and toss it all to coat well.

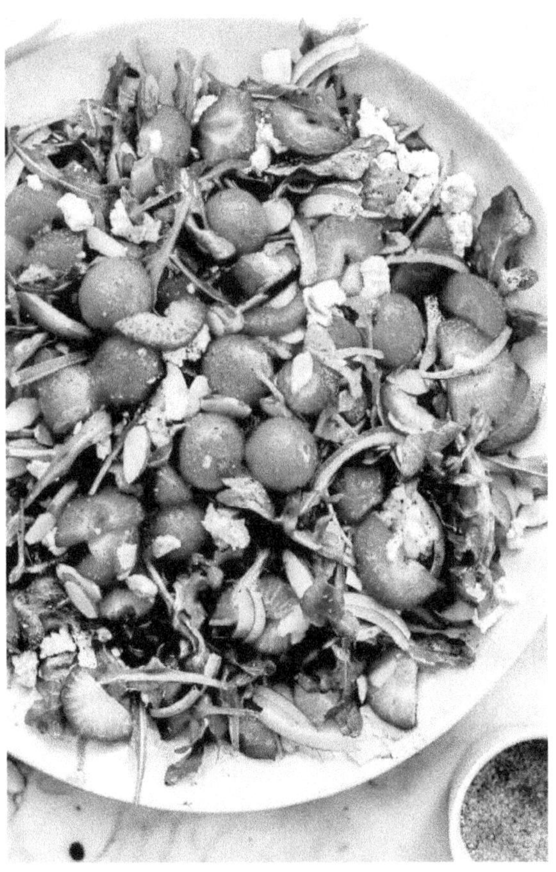

Preparation Time: 15 minutes

Cooking Time: 6 minutes

Servings: 6

Ingredients:

For Shrimp:

1 tablespoon olive oil

1 garlic clove, crushed

2 tablespoons fresh rosemary, chopped

1 pound raw shrimp, peeled and deveined

¼ teaspoon red pepper flakes, crushed

Salt and ground black pepper, as required

For Salad:

8 cups fresh arugula

3 tablespoons olive oil

2 tablespoons fresh lime juice

Salt and ground black pepper, as required

Directions:

In a large wok, heat oil over medium heat and sauté 1 garlic clove for about 1 minute. Add the shrimp with red pepper flakes, salt, and black pepper and cook for about 4-5 minutes. Remove the wok of shrimp from heat and set aside to cool. In a large bowl, add the shrimp, arugula, oil, lime juice, salt, and black pepper and gently, toss to coat. Serve immediately.

Nutrition:

Calories 182

Total Fat 11 g

Saturated Fat 1.8 g

Cholesterol 159 mg

Sodium 219 mg

Total Carbs 3.1 g

Fiber 0.9 g

Sugar 0.6 g

Protein 18 g

Preparation time: 10 Minutes

Cooking Time: 40 Minutes

Servings 4

Ingredients:

1 cup, or ¼ package if large of smoked salmon slices no cooking needed!

1 avocado, pitted, sliced, and scooped out

10 walnuts, chopped

5 lovage or celery leaves), chopped

2 celery stalks, chopped or sliced thinly

½ small red onion, sliced thinly

1 Medjool pitted date, chopped

1 tbsp. capers

1 tbsp. extra virgin olive oil

1/4 of a lemon, juiced

5 sprigs of parsley, chopped

Directions:

Wash and dry salad makings and vegetables, top with salmon.

Nutrition:

Calories 191.5 kcal

Total Fat 11.2 g

Cholesterol 48.0 mg

Sodium: 1,142.9 mg

Potassium 0.8 mg

Total Carbohydrate 2.9 g

Dietary Fiber 0.3 g

Protein 17.8 g

Preparation time: 10 Minutes

Cooking Time: 35 Minutes

Servings 4

Ingredients

10g dried wakame

1L vegetable stock

200g shiitake mushrooms, sliced

120g miso paste

1* 400g firm tofu, diced

2 green onion, trimmed and diagonally chopped

1 bird's eye chili, finely chopped

Directions

Soak the wakame in lukewarm water for 10-15 minutes before draining. In a medium-sized saucepan, add the vegetable stock and bring to the boil. Toss in the mushrooms and simmer for 2-3 minutes. Mix miso paste with 3-4 tbsp of vegetable stock from the saucepan, until the miso is entirely dissolved. Pour the miso-stock back into the pan and add the tofu, wakame, green onions, and chili, then serve immediately.

Nutrition:

Calories 137.4 kcal

Total Fat 6.7 g

Cholesterol 0.0 mg

Sodium: 1556.7 mg

Potassium: 327.6 mg

Total Carbohydrate: 11.5 g

Dietary Fiber: 2.5 g

Sugars: 3.3 g

Protein: 9.9 g

Preparation time: 10 Minutes

Cooking Time: 40 Minutes

Servings 8

Ingredients

3 garlic cloves, minced

2 cups chopped onions

1/2 cup olive oil

Salt & 1 Tsp. ground pepper to taste

4 cups vegetable broth

2 pounds dry shiitake mushrooms

Directions

Put ingredients in the slow cooker. Cover, & cook on low for 3 to 4 hours.

Nutrition:

Calories 142.2 kcal

Total Fat 2.8 g

Cholesterol 0.0 mg

Sodium: 589.2 mg

Potassium: 910.8 mg

Total Carbohydrate: 29.5 g

Dietary Fiber: 5.1 g

Sugars 4.1 g

Protein 6.0 g

Preparation time: 5 Minutes

Cooking Time: 55 Minutes

Servings 4

Ingredients

1 cup sliced leeks

1 sliced carrot

1 cup chopped onions

Salt & 1 Tsp. ground pepper to taste

2 cups chicken broth

3 cups kale

4 pounds of chicken

Directions

Put ingredients in the slow cooker. Cover, & cook on low for 7 to 9 hours.

Nutrition:

Calories 266.6 kcal

Total Fat 5.6 g

Cholesterol 49.5 mg

Sodium: 141.0 mg

Potassium: 964.2 mg

Total Carbohydrate: 33.1 g

Dietary Fiber: 8.5 g

Sugars: 4.3 g

Protein: 22.7 g

23. Fruity Granola Bars

Preparation time: 25 minutes

Cooking Time: 15 Minutes

Servings: 24 Bars

Ingredients

¾ cup packed brown sugar

½ cup honey

¼ cup of water

1 teaspoon salt

½ cup of cocoa butter

3 cups rolled oats

1 cup walnuts, chopped

1 cup ground buckwheat

¼ cup sesame seeds

½ cup dried strawberries or mixed fruits

½ cup raisins

½ cup Medjool dates, chopped

Nutrition:

Calories: 441

Fat: 17.5

Carbs:59.1

Sodium: 257

Protein: 8.7

Directions

In a large pan, combine sugar, cocoa butter, honey, water, and salt. Bring to a simmer and cook for 5 minutes. Stir in oats, walnuts, ground buckwheat, and sesame seeds. Cook, frequently stirring, for 15 minutes. Remove from heat and add dried fruits. Pour into a large baking sheet lined with wax or parchment paper. Press firmly to create an even layer. Score deeply into bars roughly 2" wide by 4" tall. Allow cooling for 30 minutes before breaking or cutting along score lines. Store in an airtight container.

Preparation time: 10 minutes

Baking time: 30 minutes

Servings: 18 Bars

Ingredients

2 cups rolled oats

½ cup raisins

½ cup walnuts, chopped and toasted

1 ½ teaspoon ground cardamom

6 tablespoons cocoa butter

1/3 cup packed brown sugar

3 tablespoons honey

Coconut oil, for greasing pan

Directions

Preheat oven to 350 degrees F. Line a 9-inch square pan with foil, extending the foil over the sides. Grease the foil with coconut oil. Mix the oats, raisins, walnuts, and cardamom in a large bowl. Heat the cocoa butter, brown sugar, and honey in a saucepan until the butter melts and begins to bubble. Pour this mixture over the dry ingredients and mix until well coated. Transfer to the prepared pan and press evenly with a spatula. Bake for 30 minutes or until the top is golden brown. Allow cooling for 30 minutes. Using the foil, lift the granola out of the pan and place on cutting board. Cut into 18 bars.

Nutrition:

Calories: 128

Fat: 6.6

Carbs: 16.7

Sodium: 30 mg

Protein: 1.9

Preparation time: 15 minutes (30 minutes – 2 hours for cooling Time)

Cooking Time: 0 Minutes

Servings: 24 – 30 Bites

Ingredients

2 ½ cups walnuts

¼ cup almonds

2 ½ cups Medjool dates

¼ cup unsweetened cocoa powder

1 teaspoon vanilla extract

¼ teaspoon of sea salt

¼ cup unsweetened desiccated or shredded coconut

Directions

Place everything in a food processor and blend until well combined. Roll into 1" balls. Roll balls in coconut until well-covered and place on a wax paper-lined baking sheet. Freeze for 30 minutes or refrigerate for up to 2 hours.

Nutrition:

Calories: 55

Fat: 6

Carbs: 6

Sodium: 5 mg

Protein: 0

Preparation time: 10 minutes

Cooking Time: 10 Minutes

Servings: 4

Ingredients

4 whole wheat flour tortillas

2 tablespoons extra virgin olive oil

4 Roma tomatoes, diced

1 small red onion, finely diced

1 Bird's Eye chili pepper, finely diced

2 teaspoons parsley, finely chopped

2 teaspoons cilantro, finely chopped

1 lime, juiced

Salt and pepper to taste

Directions

Preheat oven to 350 degrees F. Using a pastry brush, coat one side of each tortilla in olive oil. With a sharp knife or pizza cutter, divide each tortilla into 8 wedges. Spread tortillas over a large baking sheet in a single layer. Use more than one baking sheet if necessary. Bake for 8 – 10 minutes, flipping halfway through until both sides are golden brown, and your chips are crispy. While the chips are baking, combine tomatoes, red onion, chili pepper, parsley, cilantro, and lime juice and mix well. Serve salsa with the chips.

Nutrition:

Calories: 375

Fat: 19 g

Carbs: 47 g

Sodium: 215 mg

Protein: 5g

Preparation time: 30 minutes

Cooking Time: 25 Minutes

Servings: 4

Ingredients

1 bunch kale leaves

½ tablespoon extra-virgin olive oil

1 teaspoon garlic powder

1/8 teaspoon cayenne powder

¼ teaspoon fine salt

Directions

Preheat oven to 300 degrees F and cover a large baking sheet with parchment paper. Remove the stems from your kale and tear up into large pieces. Wash and spin the leaves until thoroughly dry, using a paper towel to pat dry if necessary. Place kale leaves in a large bowl and massage the olive oil thoroughly into each leaf. Combine garlic, cayenne, and salt in a small bowl and mix well. Sprinkle seasoning over kale and toss to distribute. Spread kale in a single layer over the baking sheet. Bake for 10 minutes, rotate the pan and bake for another 12-15 minutes more until the kale just begins to get crispy. The leaves will shrink and need to cool at least 5 minutes after being taken out of the oven to crisp properly.

Nutrition:

Calories: 108 kcal

Fat: 9

Carbs: 4

Sodium: 49

Protein: 2

Preparation time: 5 minutes

Cooking Time 45 minutes

Servings: 4

Ingredients

1 can of chickpeas, drained

1 - 2 tablespoon extra-virgin olive oil

½ teaspoon dried lovage

½ teaspoon dried basil

1 teaspoon garlic powder

1/8 teaspoon cayenne powder

¼ teaspoon fine salt

Directions

Preheat oven to 400 degrees F and cover a large baking sheet with parchment paper. Spread chickpeas out evenly over the pan in a single layer and roast for 30 minutes. Remove from oven and transfer to a heat-resistant bowl. Add the olive oil and toss to coat each chickpea. Sprinkle with herbs and toss again to distribute. Return to oven for an additional 15 minutes. Let cool for at least 15 minutes before eating.

Nutrition:

Calories:84

Fat: 1

Carbs: 12

Sodium: 50

Protein: 4

Preparation time: 5 minutes

Cooking Time: 20 - 25 minutes

Servings: 4

Ingredients

2 tablespoons extra virgin olive oil

½ teaspoon onion powder

½ teaspoon turmeric

½ teaspoon ground cumin

1 large head cauliflower

¾ cup shredded cheddar cheese

½ cup tomato, diced

¼ cup red bell pepper, diced

¼ cup red onion, diced

½ Bird's Eye chili pepper, finely diced

¼ cup parsley, finely diced

Pinch of salt

Directions

Preheat oven to 400 degrees F. Mix onion powder, cumin, turmeric, and olive oil. Core cauliflower and slice into ½" thick rounds. Coat the cauliflower with the olive oil mixture and bake for 15 – 20 minutes. Top with shredded cheese & bake for an additional 3 – 5 minutes, until cheese is melted. In a bowl, combine tomatoes, bell pepper, onion, chili, and parsley with a pinch of salt. Top cooked cauliflower with salsa and serve.

Nutrition:

Calories: 418.4

Fat: 26.7

Carbs: 24.7

Sodium: 453. 3

Protein: 24.8

30. Kale White Bean Pork Soup

Preparation Time: 5 Minutes

Cooking Time: 45 Minutes

Servings: 4

Ingredients:

3 tbsp extra-virgin olive oil

3 tbsp chili powder

1 tbsp jalapeno hot sauce

2 pounds bone-in pork chops

Salt

4 stalks celery, chopped

1 large white onion, chopped

3 cloves garlic, chopped

2 cups chicken broth

2 cups diced tomatoes

2 cups cooked white beans

6 cups packed kale

Nutrition:

Calories: 140

Fat: 6

Carbs: 14

Sodium: 600 mg

Protein: 7

Directions:

Preheat the broiler. Whisk hot sauce, 1 tbsp olive oil, and chili powder in a bowl. Season the pork chops with ½ tsp salt. Rub chops with the spice mixture on both sides and place them on a rack set over a baking sheet. Set aside. Heat 1 tbsp olive oil in a pot over medium heat. Add the celery, garlic, onion, and the remaining 2 tbsp chili powder. Cook until onions are translucent, stirring (approx. 8 minutes). Add tomatoes and the chicken broth to the pot. Cook and occasionally stir until reduced by about one-third (approx. 7 minutes). Add the kale and the beans. Reduce the heat to medium, cover, and cook until the kale is tender (approx. 7 minutes). Add up to ½ cup of water if the mixture looks dry and season with salt. In the meantime, boil the pork until browned (approx. 4 to 6 minutes). Flip and broil until cooked through. Serve with the kale and beans.

Preparation Time: 5 Minutes

Cooking Time: 30 Minutes

Servings: 3

Ingredients:

250g (9oz) turkey breast, cubed

25g (1oz) smooth peanut butter

1 clove of garlic, crushed

½ small bird's eye chili (or more if you like it hotter), finely chopped

½ tsp ground turmeric

200ml (7fl oz) coconut milk

2 tsp soy sauce

Nutrition:

Calories: 107

Fat: 1

Carbs: 3

Protein: 20

Directions:

Combine the coconut milk, peanut butter, turmeric, soy sauce, garlic, and chili. Add the turkey pieces to the bowl and stir them until they are completely coated. Push the turkey onto metal skewers. Place the satay skewers on a barbeque or under a hot grill (broiler) and cook for 4-5 minutes on each side, until they are completely cooked.

Preparation Time: 5
Cooking Time: 40
Servings: 3

Ingredients:

75g (3oz) Greek yogurt

4 salmon fillets, skin removed

4 tsp Dijon mustard

1 tbsp capers, chopped

2 tsp fresh parsley

Zest of 1 lemon

Directions:

In a bowl, mix together the yogurt, mustard, lemon zest, parsley, and capers. Thoroughly coat the salmon in the mixture. Place the salmon under a hot grill (broiler) and cook for 3-4 minutes on each side or until the fish is cooked. Serve with mashed potatoes and vegetables or a large green leafy salad.

Nutrition:

Calories: 430

Fat: 24 g

Carbs: 3 g

Sodium: 860 mg

Protein: 45 g

Preparation Time: 5

Cooking Time: 20

Servings: 3

Ingredients:

250g (9oz) tinned chickpeas (garbanzo beans) drained

4 chicken breasts, cubed

4 Medjool dates halved

6 dried apricots, halved

1 red onion, sliced

1 carrot, chopped

1 tsp ground cumin

1 tsp ground cinnamon

1 tsp ground turmeric

1 bird's eye chili, chopped

600ml (1 pint) chicken stock (broth)

25g (1oz) cornflour

60ml (2fl oz) water

2 tbsp fresh coriander

Directions:

Place the chicken, chickpeas (garbanzo beans), onion, carrot, chili, cumin, turmeric, cinnamon, and stock (broth) into a large saucepan. Bring it to the boil, reduce the heat and simmer for 25 minutes. Add in the dates and apricots and simmer for 10 minutes.   In a cup, mix the cornflour together with the water until it becomes a smooth paste. Pour the mixture into the saucepan and stir until it thickens. Add in the coriander (cilantro) and mix well. Serve with buckwheat or couscous.

Nutrition:

Calories: 381.8 kcal

Fat: 10.3 g

Carbs: 40.6 g

Sodium: 2147 mg

Protein: 32.3 g

Preparation Time: 5

Cooking Time: 40

Servings: 6

Ingredients:

1 tbsp olive oil

1 large red onion

2 stalks celery, including some leaves

2 large carrots

1 bunch green onions, chopped

8 cloves garlic, minced

8 sprigs fresh parsley

6 sprigs fresh thyme

2 bay leaves

1 tsp salt

2 quarts water

Nutrition:

Calories: 10 kcal

Fat: 0

Carbs: 2

Sodium: 800 mg

Protein: 0

Directions:

Chop veggies into small chunks. Heat oil in a soup pot, add onion, scallions, celery, carrots, garlic, parsley, thyme, and bay leaves. Cook over high heat for 5 to 7 minutes, stirring occasionally. Bring to a boil and add salt. Lower heat and simmer, uncovered, for 30 minutes. Strain. Other ingredients to consider: broccoli stalk, celery root

Preparation Time: 5

Cooking Time: 50

Servings: 3

Ingredients:

4lbs. fresh chicken (wings, necks, backs, legs, bones)

2 peeled onions or 1 cup chopped leeks

2 celery stalks

1 carrot

8 black peppercorns

2 sprigs fresh thyme

2 sprigs fresh parsley

1 tsp salt

Nutrition:

Calories: 38 kcal

Fat: 1 g

Carbs: 3 g

Protein: 5

Directions:

Put cold water in a stockpot and add chicken. Bring just to a boil. Skim any foam from the surface. Add other ingredients, return just to a boil, and reduce heat to a slow simmer. Simmer for 2 hours. Let cool to warm room temperature and strain. Keep chilled and use or freeze broth within a few days. Before using, defrost and boil.

Preparation Time: 5

Cooking Time: 40

Servings: 3

Ingredients:

4-5 pounds beef bones and few veal bones

1 pound of stew meat (chuck or flank steak) cut into 2-inch chunks

Olive oil

1-2 medium red onions, peeled and quartered

1-2 large carrots, cut into 1-2-inch segments

1 celery rib, cut into 1-inch segments

2-3 cloves of garlic, unpeeled

A handful of parsley stems and leaves

1-2 bay leaves

10 peppercorns

Nutrition:

Calories: 86 kcal

Fat: 2.9 g

Protein: 6 g

Directions:

Heat oven to 375F. Rub olive oil over the stew meat pieces, carrots, and onions. Place stew meat or beef scraps, stock bones, carrots, and onions in a large roasting pan. Roast in the oven for about 45 minutes, turning everything halfway through the cooking. Place everything from the oven in a large stockpot. Pour some boiling water in the oven pan and scrape up all of the browned bits and pour all in the stockpot. Add parsley, celery, garlic, bay leaves, and peppercorns to the pot. Fill the pot with cold water, to 1-inch over the top of the bones. Bring the stockpot to a regular simmer and then reduce the heat to low, so it just barely simmers. Cover the pot loosely and let simmer low and slow for 3-4 hours. Scoop away the fat and any scum that rises to the surface once in a while. After cooking, remove the bones and vegetables from the pot. Strain the broth. Let cool to room temperature and then put in the refrigerator. The fat will solidify once the broth has chilled. Discard the fat (or reuse it) and pour the broth into a jar and freeze it.

Preparation Time: 5

Cooking Time: 30

Servings: 3

Ingredients:

450g (1lb) lean minced beef

400g (14oz) chopped tomatoes

200g (7oz) red kidney beans

2 tbsp tomato purée

2 cloves of garlic, crushed

2 red onions, chopped

2 bird's eye chilies, finely chopped

1 red pepper (bell pepper), chopped

1 stick of celery, finely chopped

1 tbsp cumin

1 tbsp turmeric

1 tbsp cocoa powder

400ml (14 fl oz) beef stock (broth)

175ml (6fl oz) red wine

1 tbsp olive oil

Directions:

Heat the oil in a large saucepan, add the onion and cook for 5 minutes. Add in the garlic, celery, chili, turmeric, and cumin and cook for 2 minutes before adding then meat then cook for another 5 minutes. Pour in the stock (broth), red wine, tomatoes, tomato purée, red pepper (bell pepper), kidney beans, and cocoa powder. Simmer on low heat for 45 minutes, keep it covered, and stirring occasionally. Serve with brown rice or buckwheat.

Nutrition:

Calories: 256 kcal

Fat: 8 g

Carbs: 21 g

Sodium: 1007 mg

Protein: 24 g

Preparation Time: 5

Cooking Time: 35

Servings: 3

Ingredients:

400g (14oz) tinned chopped tomatoes

400g (14oz) large prawns (shrimps), shelled and raw

25g (1oz) fresh coriander (cilantro) chopped

3 red onions, finely chopped

3 cloves of garlic, crushed

2 bird's eye chilies

½ tsp ground coriander (cilantro)

½ tsp turmeric

400ml (14fl oz) coconut milk

1 tbsp olive oil

Juice of 1 lime

Directions:

Place the onions, garlic, tomatoes, chilies, lime juice, turmeric, ground coriander (cilantro), chilies and half of the fresh coriander (cilantro) into a blender and blitz until you have a smooth curry paste. Heat the olive oil in a frying pan, add the pasta and cook for 2 minutes. Stir in the coconut milk and warm it thoroughly. Add the prawns (shrimps) to the paste and cook them until they have turned pink and are completely cooked. Stir in the fresh coriander (cilantro). Serve with rice.

Nutrition:

Calories: 239.6 kcal

Fat: 10.7 g

Carbs: 9.2 g

Sodium: 186.4 g

Protein: 25.3 g

Preparation Time: 5

Cooking Time: 40

Servings: 3

Ingredients:

400g (14oz) chopped tomatoes

400g (14oz) tinned cannellini beans or haricot beans

8 chicken thighs, skin removed

2 carrots, peeled and finely chopped

2 red onions, chopped

4 sticks of celery

4 large mushrooms

2 red peppers (bell peppers), de-seeded and chopped

1 clove of garlic

2 tbsp soy sauce

1 tbsp olive oil

1.75 liters (3 pints) chicken stock (broth)

Nutrition:

Calories: 209.1 kcal

Fat: 6.6 g

Carbs: 6.2 g

Sodium: 667.9 mg

Protein: 31 g

Directions:

Heat the olive oil in a saucepan, add the garlic and onions and cook for 5 minutes. Add in the chicken and cook for 5 minutes, then add the carrots, cannellini beans, celery, red peppers (bell peppers), and mushrooms. Pour in the stock (broth) soy sauce and tomatoes. Bring it to the boil, reduce the heat and simmer for 45 minutes. Serve with rice or new potatoes.

Preparation Time: 5

Cooking Time: 40

Servings:3

Ingredients:

1 skinless cod fillet

½ cup buckwheat

½ red onion, sliced

2 stalks celery, sliced

10 green beans

2 cups kale, roughly chopped

3 sprigs of parsley

1 garlic clove, finely chopped

1 pinch cayenne or ½ chili

1 tsp finely chopped fresh ginger

1 tsp Sesame seeds

2 tsp of miso

1 tbsp mirin/rice wine vinegar

1 tbsp extra virgin olive oil

1 tbsp of soy sauce

1 tsp ground turmeric

Nutrition:

Calories: 266.9 kcal

Fat: 3.9g

Carbs: 9.2g

Sodium: 543.5mg

Protein: 43.7

Directions:

Coat the cod with a mixture of the miso, mirin, and 1 tsp of the oil and set aside for 30 minutes up to one hour in the refrigerator. Heat the oven to 400F, then bake the cod for 10 minutes. Sautee the onion and stir-fry in the oil that remains along with the green beans, kale, celery, chili pepper, garlic, ginger. Sautee until the kale is wilted, but the beans and celery are tender. Add dashes of water if needed to the pan as you go. Cook the buckwheat according to the packet directions with the turmeric for 3 minutes. Add the sesame seeds, parsley, and tamari to the stir-fry and serve with the greens and fish.

41. Salmon Sirt Super Salad

Preparation Time: 10 minutes

Cooking Time: 10 minutes

Servings:1

Ingredients

50g chilies

50g chicory leaves

100g smoked salmon cuts

80g avocado, stripped, stoned and cut

40g celery, cut

20g red onion, cut

15g pecans, sliced

1 tbs escapades

1 large Medjool date, hollowed and sliced

1 tbs extra virgin olive oil

¼ lemon juice

10g parsley, sliced

10g celery leaves, sliced

Nutrition:

Calories 437 kcal

Directions

Orchestrate the salad leaves on a large plate. Combine all the rest of the ingredients and serve on the leaves.

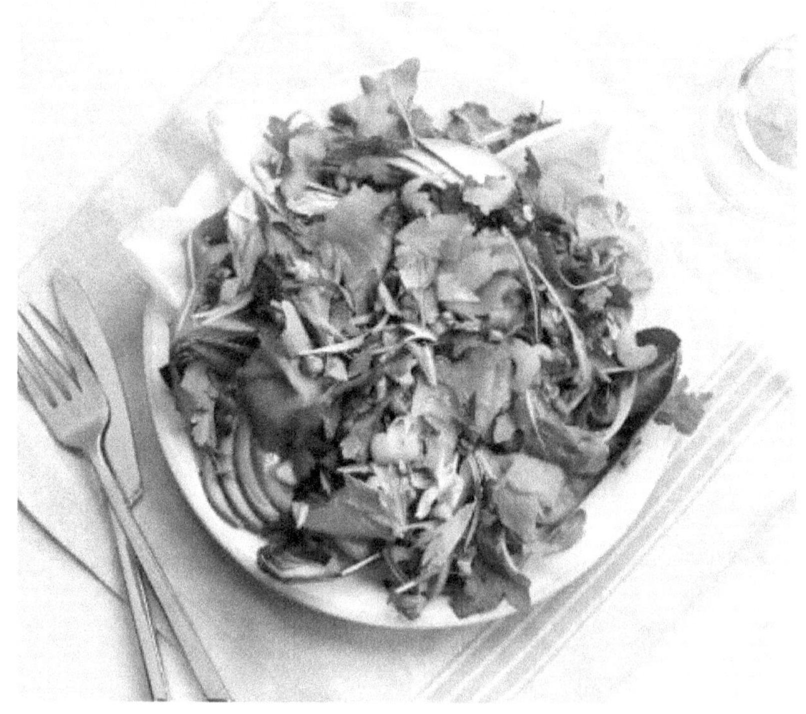

Preparation Time: 15 minutes

Cooking Time: 60 minutes

Servings: 4

Ingredients

200g oats

250g buckwheat flakes

100g walnuts, chopped

100g almonds, chopped

100g dried strawberries

1 ½ tsp ground ginger

1 ½ tsp ground cinnamon

120mls olive oil

2 tbsp honey

Directions:

Preheat oven to 150C or gas mark 3. Line a tray with baking parchment. Stir together walnuts, almonds, buckwheat flakes and oats with ginger and cinnamon. In a large pan, warm olive oil and honey, heating until the honey has dissolved. Pour the honey-oil over the other ingredients, stirring to ensuring an even coating. Separate the granola evenly over the lined baking tray and roast for 50 minutes, or until golden. Remove from the oven and leave to cool. Once cooled, add the berries and store them in an airtight container. Eat dry or with milk and yogurt. It stays fresh for up to 1 week.

Nutrition:

Calories 234

Preparation Time: 15 minutes

Cooking Time: 45 minutes

Servings: 2

Ingredients

1 tsp extra virgin olive oil

1 tsp mustard seeds

40g red onion, finely chopped

1 garlic clove, finely chopped

1 tsp finely chopped fresh ginger

1 bird's eye chili, finely chopped

1 tsp mild curry powder

2 tsp ground turmeric

300ml vegetable stock

40g red lentils, rinsed

50g kale

50ml tinned coconut milk

50g buckwheat

Directions

In a moderately sized saucepan, warm the olive oil over medium heat. Toss in the mustard seeds and fry until they start to crackle. Add the garlic, ginger, chili, and onion frying for 10 minutes, or until the onion is tender. Throw in 1 tsp turmeric and curry powder, and then stir. Cook for a few minutes until fragrant, then pour in the stock and bring to the boil. Pour in the lentils and cook for 30 minutes. Add the coconut milk and kale, cooking for another 5 minutes or so. As the dhal is brewing, rinse the buckwheat with water and cook it according to packet directions. Drain and serve with the dhal.

Nutrition:

Calories 202 kcal

Preparation Time: 10 minutes

Cooking Time: 15 minutes

Servings: 1

Ingredients

50g cheddar cheese, grated

75g kalamata olives pitted and halved

8 cherry tomatoes, halved

4 large eggs

1 tbsp fresh parsley, chopped

1 tbsp fresh basil, chopped

1 tbsp olive oil

Nutrition:

Calories: 210.8

Saturated Fat: 5.4 g

Total Fat: 13.6 g

Polyunsaturated Fat: 1.1 g

Directions

Whisk eggs together in a large mixing bowl. Toss in the parsley, basil, olives, tomatoes, and cheese, stirring thoroughly. In a small skillet, heat the olive oil over high heat. Pour in the frittata mixture and cook for 5-10 minutes, or set. Remove the skillet from the hob and place under the grill for 5 minutes, or until firm and set. Divide into portions and serve immediately.

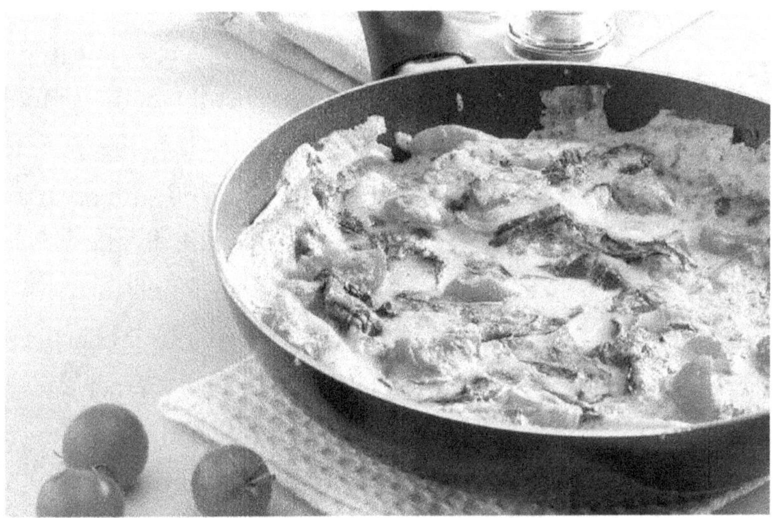

Preparation Time: 10 minutes

Cooking Time: 30 minutes

Servings: 8

Ingredients:

200g kind sized oats

50g walnuts, generally cleaved

3 tbsp light olive oil

20g margarine

1 tbsp dim darker sugar

2 tbsp rice malt syrup

60g great quality (70%)

dim chocolate chips

Directions:

Preheat the broiler to 160°C (140°C fan/Gas 3). Line an enormous heating plate with a silicone sheet or preparing material. Mix the oats and walnuts together in an enormous bowl. In a little non-stick skillet, delicately heat the olive oil, spread, dark colored sugar, and rice malt syrup until the margarine has liquefied and the sugar and syrup have broken up. Try not to permit to bubble. Pour the syrup over the oats and mix completely until the oats are completely secured. Distribute the granola over the preparing plate, spreading directly into the corners. Leave bunches of blend with separating instead of an even spread. Prepare in the broiler for 20 minutes until just tinged brilliant dark colored at the edges. Expel from the broiler and leave to cool on the plate totally. When cool, separate any greater irregularities on the plate with your fingers and afterward blend in the chocolate chips. Scoop or empty the granola into a sealed shut tub or container. The granola will keep for in any event 2 weeks.

Nutrition:

Calories 100 kcal

Preparation Time: 15 minutes

Cooking Time: 30 minutes

Servings: 1

Ingredients

200g skinless, boneless salmon fillet

50g green beans

75g kale

1 tbsp extra virgin olive oil

½ garlic clove, crushed

50g red onion, chopped

1 tbsp fresh chives, chopped

1 tbsp freshly chopped flat-leaf parsley

1 tbsp low-fat crème fraiche

1tbsp horseradish sauce

Juice of ¼ lemon

A pinch of salt and pepper

Nutrition:

Calories 265

Directions

Preheat the grill. Sprinkle a salmon fillet with salt and pepper. Place under the grill for 10-15 minutes. Flake and set aside. Using a steamer, cook the kale and green beans for 10 minutes.

In a skillet, warm the oil over high heat. Add garlic and red onion and fry for 2-3 minutes. Toss in the kale and beans, and then cook for 1-2 minutes more. Mix the chives, parsley, crème fraiche, horseradish, lemon juice, and flaked salmon. Serve the kale and beans topped with the dressed flaked salmon.

Directions Time: 15 minutes

Cooking Time: 30 minutes

Servings: 1

Ingredients

75g porridge oats

125g plain flour

1 tsp heating powder

2 tbsp caster sugar

Spot of salt

2 apples, stripped, cored and cut into little pieces

300ml semi-skimmed milk

2 egg whites

2 tsp light olive oil

For the compote:

120g blackcurrants washed and expelled

2 tbsp caster sugar

3 tbsp water

Nutrition:

Calories 289

Directions

First, make the compote. Spot the blackcurrants, sugar, and water in a little dish. Raise to a stew and cook for 10-15 minutes. Spot the oats, flour, heating powder, caster sugar and salt in a large bowl and blend well. Mix in the apple and afterward rush in the milk a little at once until you have a smooth blend. Whisk the egg whites to hardened pinnacles and afterward overlap into the flapjack player. Move the hitter to a container. Heat ½ tsp oil in a non-stick skillet on a medium-high temperature and for in roughly one-fourth of the hitter. Cook on the two sides until brilliant brown. Evacuate and rehash to make four pancakes. Serve the pancakes with the blackcurrant compote sprinkled over.

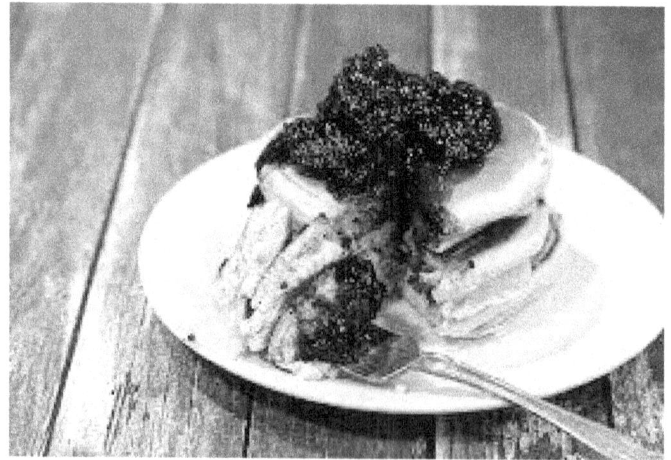

Directions Time: 15 minutes

Cooking Time: 20 minutes

Servings: 1

Ingredients

1/3 cup (50g) buckwheat

1 tablespoon ground turmeric

½ cup (80g) avocado

3/8 cup (65g) tomato

1/8 cup (20g) red onion

1/8 cup (25g) Medjool dates, pitted

1 tablespoon tricks

¾ cup (30g) parsley

2/3 cup (100g) strawberries, hulled

1 tablespoon extra-virgin olive oil

juice of ½ lemon

1 ounce (30g) arugula

.

Directions

Cook the buckwheat with the turmeric as per the bundle Directions. Channel and put aside to cool.

Finely cleave the avocado, tomato, red onion, dates, escapades, and parsley and blend in with the cool buckwheat. Cut the strawberries and delicately blend into the plate of salad with the oil and lemon juice. Serve on a bed of arugula

Nutrition:
Calories 189 kcal

Preparation Time: 10 minutes

Cooking Time: 10 minutes

Servings: 1

Ingredients

50g buckwheat pasta (cooked)

large bunch of chilies

a little bunch of basil leaves

8 cherry tomatoes, divided

½ avocado, diced

10 olives

1 tbsp extra virgin olive oil

20g pine nuts

Nutrition:

Calories 220

Fat: 3g

Carbs: 40 g

Sodium: 2070 mg

Protein 7g

Directions

Delicately combine all the ingredients aside from the pine nuts and organize on a plate or in a bowl; at that point, dissipate the pine nuts over the top.

50. Tuscan Bean Stew

Preparation Time: 15 minutes

Cooking Time: 40 minutes

Servings: 1

Ingredients

1 tbsp extra virgin olive oil

50g red onion, finely sliced

30g carrot, stripped and finely sliced

30g celery, cut and finely sliced

1 garlic slice, finely sliced

½ 10,000 foot bean stew, finely sliced (optional)

1 tsp Provence herbs

200ml vegetable stock

1 x 400g tin sliced Italian tomatoes

1 tsp tomato puree

200g tinned blended beans

50g kale, generally sliced

1 tbsp generally sliced parsley

40g buckwheat

Nutrition:

Calories 382

Directions

Spot the oil in a medium pot over low – medium heat and delicately fry the onion, carrot, celery, garlic, bean stew (if utilizing) and herbs, until the onion is delicate, however not shaded. Include the stock, tomatoes and tomato purée and bring to the bubble. Include the beans and stew for 30 minutes. Include the kale and cook for another 5–10 minutes until delicate, at that point, include the parsley. In the interim, cook the buckwheat as indicated by the bundle Directions, channel, and afterward present with the stew.

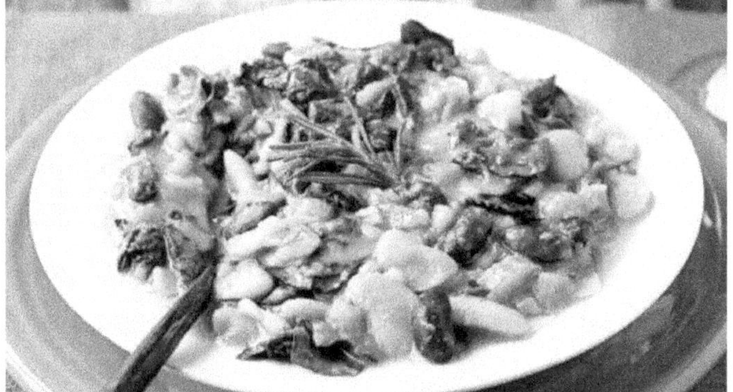

Preparation Time: 10 minutes

Cooking Time: 15 minutes

Servings: 1

Ingredients

400g firm tofu, cut into huge blocks

1 tbsp cornflour Sirtfood recipe

1 tbsp water

125ml chicken stock

1 tbsp rice wine

1 tbsp tomato puree

1 tsp brown sugar

1 tbsp soy sauce

1 slice garlic, stripped and squashed

1 thumb ginger, stripped and ground

1 tbsp rapeseed oil

100g shiitake mushrooms, cut

1 shallot, stripped and cut

200g pak choi or choi whole, cut into slim cuts

400g slender pork (10% fat)

100g beansprouts

Large quantity (20g) parsley, sliced

Nutrition:

Calories 481 Kcal

Directions

Spread out the tofu on kitchen paper, spread with more kitchen paper and put in a safe spot.

In a little bowl, combine the cornflour and water, expelling all irregularities. Include the chicken stock, rice wine, tomato puree, brown sugar, and soy sauce. Include the squashed garlic and ginger and mix together. In a wok or huge pan, heat the oil to at high temperature. Include the shiitake mushrooms and pan-fried food for 2–3 minutes until cooked and lustrous. Expel the mushrooms from the dish with an opened spoon and put it in a safe spot. Add the tofu to the skillet and pan-fried food until brilliant on all sides. Evacuate with an opened spoon and put it in a safe spot. Include the shallot and pak choi to the wok, pan sear for 2 minutes, at that point, include the mince. Cook until the mince is cooked through; at that point, include the sauce, decrease the heat an indent and permit the sauce to rise round the meat for a moment or two. Include the beansprouts, shiitake mushrooms, and tofu to the container and heat through. Expel from the heat, mix through the parsley, and serve right away

Preparation Time: 15 minutes

Cooking Time: 45 minutes

Servings: 1

Ingredients

2 tablespoons olive oil

1 red onion, cut

2cm ginger, ground

3 garlic slices, ground or squashed

1 teaspoon stew pieces (or to taste)

2 teaspoons cumin seeds

1 cinnamon stick

2 ground turmeric teaspoons

800g lamb neck filet, cut into 2cm pieces

½ teaspoon salt

100g Medjool dates, hollowed and sliced

400g tin sliced tomatoes, in addition to a large portion of a jar of water

500g butternut squash, sliced into 1cm solid shapes

400g tin chickpeas, depleted

2 tablespoons new coriander

Buckwheat, couscous, flatbreads or rice to serve

Nutrition:

Calories 431

Directions

Preheat your stove to 140C. Drizzle around 2 tablespoons of olive oil into a huge ovenproof pot or cast-iron goulash dish. Include the cut onion and cook on a delicate heat, with the top on, for around 5 minutes, until the onions are cooked, yet not brown. Add the grounded garlic and ginger, bean stew, cumin, cinnamon, and turmeric. Mix well and cook for 1 progressively minute with the cover off. Include a sprinkle of water on the off chance that it gets excessively dry. Next, include the lamb lumps. Mix well to cover the meat in the onions and flavors and afterward include the salt, sliced dates, and tomatoes, in addition to about a large portion of a container of water (100-200ml). Bring the tagine to boil and afterward put the top on and put in your preheated stove for 1 hour and 15 minutes. Thirty minutes before the finish of the cooking time, include the sliced butternut squash and depleted chickpeas. Mix everything together, set the cover back on, and come back to the stove for the last 30 minutes of cooking. When the tagine is prepared, expel from the stove and mix through the sliced coriander. Present with buckwheat, couscous, flatbreads, or basmati rice.

53. Chargrilled Beef with A Red Wine Jus, Onion Rings, Garlic Kale, and Herb Simmered Potatoes

Preparation Time: 15 minutes

Cooking Time: 30 minutes

Servings: 1

Ingredients

100g potatoes, stripped and cut into 2cm shakers

1 tbsp extra virgin olive oil

5g parsley, finely sliced

50g red onion, cut into rings

50g kale, cut

1 garlic slice, finely sliced

120–150g x 3.5cm-thick hamburger filet steak or 2cm-thick sirloin steak

40ml red wine

150ml hamburger stock

1 tsp tomato puree

1 tsp cornflour, broke down in 1 tbsp water

Directions

Heat the broiler to 220°C/gas 7. Spot the potatoes in a pan of bubbling water, take back to the bubble and cook for 4–5 minutes, at that point channel. Spot in a broiling tin with 1 teaspoon of the oil and dish in the hot broiler for 35–45 minutes. Turn the potatoes like clockwork to guarantee in any event, cooking. At the point when cooked, expel from the broiler, sprinkle with the sliced parsley, and blend well. Fry the onion in 1 teaspoon of the oil over medium heat for 5–7 minutes, until delicate and pleasantly caramelized. Keep warm. Steam the kale for 2–3 minutes at that point channel. Fry the garlic tenderly in ½ teaspoon of oil for 1 moment, until delicate however not colored. Include the kale and fry for a further 1–2 minutes, until delicate. Keep warm. Heat an ovenproof skillet over high temperature until smoking. Coat the meat in ½ a teaspoon of the oil and fry in the hot skillet over a medium-high temperature as indicated by how you like your meat done. If you like your meat medium, it is smarter to burn the meat and afterward move the dish to a stove set at 220°C/gas 7 and finish the cooking that path for the endorsed occasions.

Expel the meat from the dish and put aside to rest. Add the wine to the hot container to raise any meat buildup. Air pocket to decrease the wine considerably, until sweet and with a concentrated flavor. Include the stock and tomato purée to the steak skillet and bring it to the bubble. At that point, add the cornflour glue to thicken your sauce, including it a little at once, until you have your ideal consistency. Mix in any of the juices from the refreshed steak and present with the broiled potatoes, kale, onion rings, and red wine sauce.

Nutrition:
Calories 473 kcal

Preparation Time: 15 minutes

Cooking Time: 15 minutes

Servings: 1

Ingredients

125-150 g Skinned Salmon

1 tsp Extra virgin olive oil

1 tsp ground turmeric

1/4 Juice of a lemon

For the fiery celery

1 tsp Extra virgin olive oil

40 g Red onion, finely slashed

60 g Tinned green lentils

1 Garlic clove, finely slashed

1 cm fresh ginger, finely slashed

1 Bird's eye bean stew, finely slashed

150 g Celery, cut into 2cm lengths

1 tsp Mild curry powder

130 g Tomato, cut into 8 wedges

100 ml Chicken or vegetable stock

1 tbsp Chopped parsley

Nutrition:

Calories 324

Directions

Heat the broiler to 200C/gas mark 6.

Start with the hot celery. Warmth a griddle over medium-low warmth, include the olive oil, then the onion, garlic, ginger, bean stew, and celery. Fry delicately for 2–3 minutes or until softened; however not hued, then include the curry powder and cook for a further moment.

Add the tomatoes, then the stock and lentils, and stew tenderly for 10 minutes. You might need to increment or diminishing the cooking time contingent upon how crunchy you like your celery. Meanwhile, blend the turmeric, oil, and lemon squeeze and rub over the salmon. # Place on a heating plate and cook for 8–10 minutes.

To complete, mix the parsley through the celery and present it with the salmon.

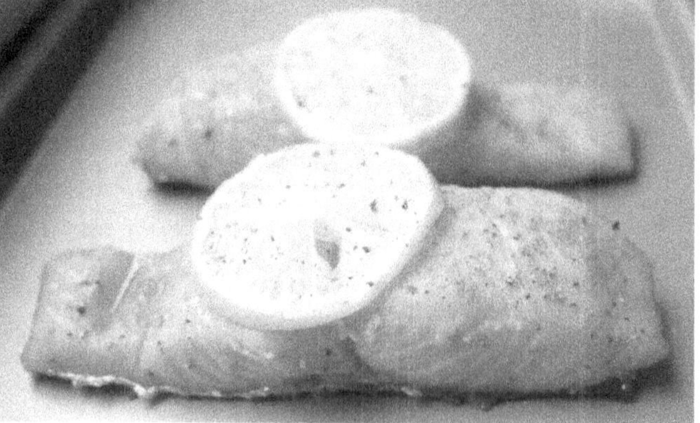

Preparation Time: 15 minutes

Cooking Time: 45 minutes

Servings: 1

Ingredients

75g brown rice

1 pak choi

60ml chicken stock

1 tbsp extra virgin olive oil

1 garlic clove, finely chopped

50g red onion, finely chopped

½ bird's eye chili, finely chopped

1 tsp freshly grated ginger

125g shelled raw king prawns

1 tbsp soy sauce

1 tsp five-spice

1 tbsp freshly chopped flat-leaf parsley

A pinch of salt and pepper

Directions

Bring a medium-sized saucepan of water to the boil and cook the brown rice for 25-30 minutes, or until softened. Tear the pak choi into pieces. Warm the chicken stock in a skillet over medium heat and toss in the pak choi, cooking until the pak choi has slightly wilted. In another skillet, warm olive oil over high heat. Toss in the ginger, chili, red onions and garlic frying for 2-3 minutes. Throw in the pawns, five-spice and soy sauce and cook for 6-8 minutes, or until the cooked throughout. Drain the brown rice and add to the skillet, stirring and cooking for 2-3 minutes. Add the pak choi, garnish with parsley and serve.

Nutrition:

Calories: 484 kcal

Fat 20g

Saturates 3g

Carbs 48g

Sugars 9g

Fiber 7g

Protein 25g

56. Tuna Salad

Preparation Time: 10 minutes

Cooking Time: 10 minutes

Servings: 2

Ingredients

100g red chicory

150g tuna flakes in brine, drained

100g cucumber

25g rocket

6 kalamata olives, pitted

2 hard-boiled eggs, peeled and quartered

2 tomatoes, chopped

2 tbsp fresh parsley, chopped

1 red onion, chopped

1 celery stalk

1 tbsp capers

2 tbsp garlic vinaigrette

Directions

Combine all ingredients in a bowl and serve.

Nutrition:

Calories 251

Preparation Time: 10 minutes

Cooking Time: 15 minutes

Servings: 1

Ingredients

250g kale, finely chopped

50g walnuts, chopped

75g feta cheese, broken

1 apple, peeled, cored & diced

4 Medjool dates, chopped

75g cranberries

½ red onion, chopped

3 tbsp olive oil

3 tbsp water

2 tsp honey

1 tbsp red wine vinegar

A pinch of salt

Nutrition:

Calories: 186.4

Fiber: 2.5 g

Sodium: 475.9 mg

Directions

In a bowl, throw together the kale, walnuts, feta cheese, apple, and dates, and then stir.

In a food processor, add cranberries, red onion, olive oil, water, honey, red wine vinegar, and a pinch of salt. Process until smooth and fluid, adding water if necessary. Pour the cranberry dressing over the salad and serve.

Preparation Time: 10 minutes

Cooking Time: 10 minutes

Servings: 1

Ingredients

50g buckwheat pasta sirtfood plans

enormous bunch of rockets

a little bunch of basil leaves

8 cherry tomatoes, halved

1/2 avocado, diced

10 olives

1 tbsp additional virgin olive oil

20g pine nuts

Nutrition:

Calories 247

Directions:

Delicately join every one of the ingredients aside from the pine nuts and orchestrate on a plate or in a bowl, then dissipate the pine nuts over the top.

Preparation Time: 15 minutes

Cooking Time: 30 minutes

Servings: 2

Ingredients

1 tbsp sesame seeds

1 cucumber, stripped, split lengthways, deseeded with a teaspoon and cut

100g child kale, generally cleaved

60g pak choi, finely destroyed

½ red onion, finely cut

Huge bunch (20g) parsley, cleaved

150g cooked chicken, destroyed

For the dressing:

1 tbsp additional virgin olive oil

1 tsp sesame oil

Juice of 1 lime

1 tsp clear nectar

2 tsp soy sauce

Directions:

Toast the sesame seeds in a dry griddle for 2 minutes until delicately sautéed and fragrant. Move to a plate to cool. In a little bowl, combine the olive oil, sesame oil, lime juice, nectar, and soy sauce to make the dressing. Place the cucumber, kale, pak choi, red onion, and parsley in a huge bowl and delicately combine. Pour over the dressing and blend once more. Distribute the serving of mixed greens between two plates and top with the destroyed chicken. Sprinkle over the sesame seeds just before serving.

Nutrition:

Calories 329 kcal

Fat: 18 g

Carbs: 34.7 g

Fiber: 7.6 g

Protein: 24.1 g

Preparation Time: 15 minutes

Cooking Time: 25 minutes

Servings: 1

Ingredients:

½ cup crisply made green tea

1 tsp nectar

1 orange, divided

1 apple, cored and generally slashed

10 red seedless grapes

10 blueberries

Direction

1 Stir the nectar into a large portion of some green tea. When broken down, include the juice of a large portion of the orange. Leave to cool.

2 Chop the other portion of the orange and spot in a bowl together with the cleaved apple, grapes, and blueberries. Pour over the cooled tea and leave to soak for a couple of moments before serving.

Nutrition:

Calories 234 kcal

Preparation Time: 5 minutes

Cooking Time: 10 minutes

Servings: 1

Ingredients:

75 g Natural yogurt

Juice of 1/4 of a lemon

1 tsp Coriander, cleaved

1 tsp ground turmeric

1/2 tsp Mild curry powder

100 g Cooked chicken bosom, cut into scaled-down pieces

6 Walnut parts, finely slashed

1 Medjool date, finely slashed

20 g Red onion, diced

1 Bird's eye bean stew

40 g Rocket, to serve

Directions

Blend the yogurt, lemon juice, coriander, and flavors together in a bowl. Include all the rest of the ingredients and serve on a bed of the rocket.

Nutrition:

Calories 314

Preparation Time: 15 Minutes

Cooking Time: 15 Minutes

Servings: 1

Ingredients:

1 3/4 ounces (50g) arugula

1 3/4 ounces (50g) endive leaves

3 1/2 ounces (100g) smoked salmon cuts

1/2 cup (80g) avocado, stripped, stoned, and cut

1/2 cup (50g) celery including leaves, cut

1/8 cup (20g) red onion, cut

1/8 cups (15g) pecans, slashed

1 tablespoon escapades

1 enormous Medjool date, hollowed and slashed

1 tablespoon additional virgin olive oil

juice of 1/4 lemon

1/4 cup (10g) parsley, slashed

Directions:

Spot the serving of mixed greens on a plate or in an enormous bowl. Combine all the rest of the ingredients and serve over the leaves.

Nutrition:

Calories 236

63. Asian king prawn stir-fry with buckwheat noodles

Preparation Time: 10 minutes

Cooking Time: 20 minutes

Servings: 1

Ingredients

150g shelled raw ruler prawns

2 tsp tamari

2 tsp extra virgin olive oil

75g soba

1 garlic slice

1 elevated stew

1 tsp sliced ginger

20g red onions

40g celery

75g green beans

50g kale

100ml chicken stock

5g celery leaves

Nutrition:

Calories 402

Directions

Heat a pan over, at that point, cook the prawns in 1 teaspoon of the tamari and 1 teaspoon of the oil for 2–3 minutes. Move the prawns to a plate. Wipe the work out with kitchen paper, as you're going to utilize it once more. Cook the noodles in bubbling water for 5–8 minutes or as coordinated on the parcel. Channel and put in a safe spot. Then, fry the garlic, stew and ginger, red onion, celery, beans, and kale in the rest of the oil over medium-high temperature for 2–3 minutes. Add the stock and bring to the bubble, at that point stew for a moment or two, until the vegetables are cooked yet at the same time crunchy.

Include the prawns, noodles, and lovage/celery leaves to the skillet, take back to the bubble at that point expel from the heat and serve.

Preparation Time: 10 minutes

Cooking Time: 15 minutes

Servings: 1

Ingredients

2 wooden sticks, absorbed water for 30 minutes before use

8 large dark olives

8 cherry tomatoes

1 yellow pepper, cut into 8 squares

½ red onion cut down the middle and isolated into 8 pieces

100g (about 10cm) cucumber, cut into 4 cuts and divided

100g feta, cut into 8 solid shapes

For the dressing:

1 tbsp extra virgin olive oil

Juice of ½ lemon

1 tsp balsamic vinegar

½ slice garlic, stripped and squashed

Directions

Add leaves basil, finely sliced (or ½ tsp dried blended herbs to supplant basil and oregano)

Add oregano leaves, finely sliced

Liberal flavoring of salt and newly ground dark pepper

String each stick with the plate of salad Ingredients in the request: olive, tomato, yellow pepper, red onion, cucumber, feta, tomato, olive, yellow pepper, red onion, cucumber, feta.

Spot all the dressing ingredients in a little bowl and combine them all together for over the sticks.

Nutrition:

Calories 329

Preparation Time: 10 minutes

Cooking Time: 20 minutes

Servings: 1

Ingredients

150g cauliflower, roughly chopped

1 garlic clove, finely chopped

40g red onion, finely chopped

1 bird's eye chili, finely chopped

1 tsp finely chopped fresh ginger

2 tbsp extra virgin olive oil

2 tsp ground turmeric

30g sun-dried tomatoes, finely chopped

10g parsley

150g turkey steak

1 tsp dried sage

Juice of ½ lemon

1 tbsp capers

Directions

Disintegrate the cauliflower using a food processor. Blend in 1-2 pulses until the cauliflower has a breadcrumb-like consistency. In a skillet, fry garlic, chili, ginger, and red onion in 1 tsp olive oil for 2-3 minutes. Throw in the turmeric and cauliflower then cook for another 1-2 minutes. Remove from heat and add the tomatoes and roughly half the parsley. Garnish the turkey steak with sage and dress with oil. In a skillet, over medium heat, fry the turkey steak for 5 minutes, turning occasionally. Once the steak is cooked, add lemon juice, capers, and a dash of water. Stir and serve with the couscous.

Nutrition:

Calories 394

Preparation Time: 10 minutes

Cooking Time: 35 minutes

Servings: 1

Ingredients

1 tbsp mirin

20g miso paste

1 * 150g firm tofu

40g celery, trimmed

35g red onion

120g courgette

1 bird's eye chili

1 garlic clove, finely chopped

1 tsp finely chopped fresh ginger

50g kale, chopped

2 tsp sesame seeds

35g buckwheat

1 tsp ground turmeric

2 tsp extra virgin olive oil

1 tsp tamari (or soy sauce)

Directions

Pre-heat your over to 200C or gas mark 6. Cover a tray with baking parchment. Combine the mirin and miso together. Dice the tofu and coat it in the mirin-miso mixture in a resealable plastic bag. Set aside to marinate. Chop the vegetables (except for the kale) at a diagonal angle to produce long slices. Using a steamer, cook for the kale for 5 minutes and set aside. Disperse the tofu across the lined tray and garnish with sesame seeds. Roast for 20 minutes, or until caramelized. Rinse the buckwheat using running water and a sieve. Add to a pan of boiling water alongside turmeric and cook the buckwheat according to the packet Directions. Heat the oil in a skillet over high heat. Toss in the vegetables, herbs, and spices, then fry for 2-3 minutes. Reduce to medium heat and fry for a further 5 minutes or until cooked but still crunchy.

Nutrition:
Calories 273

Preparation Time: 10 minutes

Cooking Time: 25 minutes

Servings: 2

Ingredients

150g shelled raw king prawns, deveined

2 tsp tamari

2 tsp extra virgin olive oil

75 soba

1 garlic clove, finely chopped

1 bird's eye chili, finely chopped

1 tsp finely chopped fresh ginger

20g red onions, sliced

40g celery, trimmed and sliced

75g green beans, chopped

50g kale, roughly chopped

100ml chicken stock

Directions

Warm a skillet over high heat, and then fry for the pawns in 1 tbsp of the tamari and 1 tsp of olive oil. Transfer the contents of the skillet to a plate and then wipe the skillet with a kitchen towel to remove the lingering sauce. Boil water and cook the soba for 8 minutes, or according to packet directions. Drain and set aside for later. Using the remaining 1 tsp olive oil, fry the remaining ingredients for 3-4 minutes. Add the stock and bring to the boil, simmering until the vegetables are tender but still have a bite. Add the lovage, noodles, and prawn into the skillet, stir, bring back to the boil and then serve.

Nutrition:

Calories 435 kcal

Preparation Time: 10 minutes

Cooking Time: 20 minutes

Servings: 1

Ingredients

100g tofu, extra firm

1 tsp ground turmeric

1 tsp mild curry powder

20g kale, roughly chopped

1 tsp extra virgin olive oil

20g red onion, thinly sliced

50g mushrooms, thinly sliced

5g parsley, finely chopped

Directions

Place 2 sheets of kitchen towel under and on top of the tofu, then rest a considerable weight such as saucepan onto the tofu, to ensure it drains off the liquid.

Combine the curry powder, turmeric, and 1-2 tsp of water to form a paste. Using a steamer cook kale for 3-4 minutes.

In a skillet, warm oil over medium heat. Add the chili, mushrooms, and onion, cooking for several minutes or until brown and tender.

Break the tofu into small pieces and toss in the skillet. Coat with the spice paste and stir, ensuring everything becomes evenly coated. Cook for up to 5 minutes, or until the tofu has browned, then add the kale and fry for 2 more minutes. Garnish with parsley before serving.

Nutrition:

Calories 131

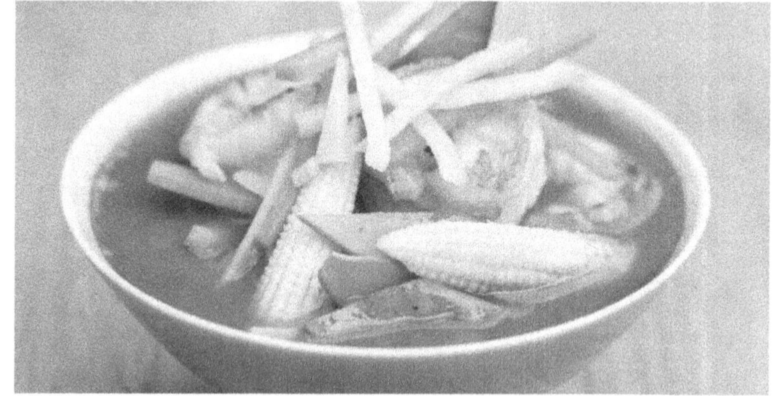

Preparation Time: 10 minutes

Cooking Time: 15 minutes

Servings: 2

Ingredients:

1 tsp tomato purée

1 star anise, squashed (or 1/4 tsp ground anise)

Little bunch (10g) parsley, stalks finely cleaved

Little bunch (10g) coriander, stalks finely cleaved

Juice of 1/2 lime

500ml chicken stock, new or made with 1 solid shape

1/2 carrot, stripped and cut into matchsticks

50g broccoli, cut into little florets

50g beansprouts

100 g crude tiger prawns

100 g firm tofu, slashed

50g rice noodles, cooked according to parcel directions

50g cooked water chestnuts, depleted

20g sushi ginger, slashed

1 tbsp great quality miso glue

Nutrition:

Calories 434

Directions:

Spot the tomato purée, star anise, parsley stalks, coriander stalks, lime juice, and chicken stock in an enormous container and bring to a stew for 10 minutes. Include the carrot, broccoli, prawns, tofu, noodles, and water chestnuts and stew tenderly until the prawns are cooked through. Expel from the warmth and mix in the sushi ginger and miso glue. Serve sprinkled with the parsley and coriander leaves.

Preparation Time: 15 minutes

Cooking Time: 30 minutes

Servings: 2

Ingredients

2 wooden sticks, absorbed water for 30 minutes before use

8 enormous dark olives

8 cherry tomatoes

1 yellow pepper, cut into 8 squares

½ red onion, cut down the middle and isolated into 8 pieces

100g (about 10cm) cucumber, cut into 4 cuts and divided

100g feta, cut into 8 shapes

For the dressing:

1 tbsp additional virgin olive oil

Juice of ½ lemon

1 tsp balsamic vinegar

½ clove garlic, stripped and squashed

Scarcely any departs basil, finely hacked (or ½ tsp dried blended herbs to supplant basil and oregano)

leaves oregano, finely slashed

Liberal flavoring of salt and crisply ground dark pepper

Nutrition:

Calories 364

Directions:

Thread each stick with the plate of mixed greens ingredients in the request: olive, tomato, yellow pepper, red onion, cucumber, feta, tomato, olive, yellow pepper, red onion, cucumber, feta. Place all the dressing ingredients in a little bowl and combine them all together. Pour over the sticks.

Preparation Time: 15 Minutes

Cooking Time: 35 Minutes

Servings: 2

Ingredients

120g skinless, boneless chicken bosom

2 tsp ground turmeric

juice of ¼ lemon

1 tbsp additional virgin olive oil

50g kale slashed

20g red onion, cut

1 tsp slashed new ginger

50g buckwheat

Nutrition:

Calories 465

Directions:

To make the salsa, expel the eye from the tomato and slash it finely, taking consideration to keep however much of the fluid as could reasonably be expected. Blend in with the bean stew, tricks, parsley, and lemon juice. You could place everything in a blender, yet the final product is somewhat different. Warm the broiler to 220°C/gas 7. Marinate the chicken bosom in 1 teaspoon of the turmeric, the lemon juice, and a little oil. Leave for 5–10 minutes. Warmth an ovenproof griddle until hot, then include the marinated chicken and cook for a moment or so on each side, until pale brilliant, then exchange to the broiler (place on a preparing plate if your skillet isn't ovenproof) for 8–10 minutes or until cooked through. Expel from the broiler, spread with foil and leave to rest for 5 minutes before serving. In the meantime, cook the kale in a steamer for 5 minutes. Fry the red onions and the ginger in a little oil, until delicate however not shaded, then include the cooked kale and fry for one more moment. Cook the buckwheat according to the parcel Directions with the rest of the teaspoon of turmeric. Serve nearby the chicken, vegetables, and salsa.

Preparation Time: 15 minutes

Cooking Time: 40 minutes

Servings: 1

Ingredients

1 tbsp additional virgin olive oil

50g red onion, finely hacked

30g carrot, stripped and finely chopped

30g celery, cut and finely hacked

1 garlic clove, finely hacked

½ 10,000 foot bean stew, finely slashed (discretionary)

1 tsp herbs de Provence

200ml vegetable stock

1 x 400g tin hacked Italian tomatoes

1 tsp tomato purée

200g tinned blended beans

50g kale, generally hacked

1 tbsp generally hacked parsley

40g buckwheat

Directions

Spot the oil in a medium pot over a low–medium warmth and delicately fry the onion, carrot, celery, garlic, chili (if utilizing) and herbs, until the onion is delicate yet not shaded. Include the stock, tomatoes and tomato purée and bring to the bubble. Include the beans and stew for 30 minutes. Include the kale and cook for another 5–10 minutes, until delicate, then include the parsley. In the interim, cook the buckwheat according to the bundle Directions, deplete, and afterward present with the stew.

Nutrition:

Calories 289

73. Sirtfood bites

Preparation Time: 10 Minutes

Cooking Time: 0 Minutes

Servings: 15-20

Ingredients:

1 cup pecans

1 ounce dull chocolate, broken into pieces; or 1/4 cup cocoa nibs

9 ounces Medjool dates, pitted

1 tablespoon cocoa powder

1 tablespoon ground turmeric

1 tablespoon additional virgin olive oil

the scratched seeds of 1 vanilla unit or 1 teaspoon vanilla concentrate

1 to 2 tablespoons of water

Directions:

Spot the pecans and chocolate in a nourishment processor and procedure until you have a fine powder. Include the various Ingredients aside from the water and mix until the blend frames a ball. You could conceivably need to include the water depending on the consistency of the blend—you don't need it to be excessively clingy. Utilizing your hands, structure the blend into reduced down balls and refrigerate in a water/air proof compartment for at any rate 1 hour before eating them. You could move a portion of the balls in some more cocoa or dried coconut to accomplish a different completion if you like. They will keep for as long as multi-week in your ice chest.

Nutrition:

Calories 202

Preparation Time: 15 minutes

Cooking Time: 15 minutes

Servings: 1

Ingredients:

20g buckwheat flakes

10g buckwheat puffs

15g coconut drops or dried up coconut

40g Medjool dates, hollowed and slashed

15g pecans, slashed

10g cocoa nibs

100g strawberries, hulled and slashed

100g plain Greek yogurt (or vegetarian elective, for example, soya or coconut yogurt)

Directions:

Blend the entire ingredients together, possibly including the yogurt and strawberries before serving if you are making it in mass.

Nutrition:

Calories 200

Preparation Time: 15 minutes

Cooking Time: 50 minutes

Servings: 2

Ingredients:

100g raspberries, washed

2 leaves gelatin

100g blackcurrants, washed and stalks evacuated

2 tbsp granulated sugar

300ml water

Directions:

Arrange the raspberries in two serving dishes/glasses/molds. Put the gelatine leaves in a bowl of cold water to soften. Place the blackcurrants in a little container with the sugar and 100ml water and bring it to the bubble. Stew vivaciously for 5 minutes and afterward expel from the warmth. Leave to represent 2 minutes. Squeeze out overabundance water from the gelatine leaves and add them to the pot. Mix until completely broken up, then mix in the remainder of the water. Empty the fluid into the readied dishes and refrigerate to set. The jams ought to be prepared in around 3-4 hours or medium-term.

Nutrition:

Calories 142

Fat: 0.22 g

Carbs: 15.5 g

Sodium: 1.1 mg

Protein: 1.6 g

Preparation Time: 5 Minutes

Cooking Time: 10 Minutes

Servings: 1

Ingredients

2 eggs

1 tsp ground turmeric

1 tsp gentle curry powder

20g kale, generally hacked

1 tsp additional virgin olive oil

½ 10,000 foot bean stew, daintily cut

bunch of catch mushrooms, daintily cut

5g parsley, finely slashed

Seed blend as a topper and some Rooster Sauce for enhancing (optional)

Nutrition:

Calories 235

Directions

Blend the turmeric and curry powder and include a little water until you have accomplished a light glue. Steam the kale for 2–3 minutes. Warmth the oil in a griddle over medium warmth and fry the stew and mushrooms for 2–3 minutes until they have begun to dark-colored and soften.

Preparation Time: 10 minutes

Cooking Time: 15 minutes

Servings: 1

Ingredients

1 tsp extra virgin olive oil

20g red onion, finely chopped

½ bird's eye chili, finely chopped

3 medium eggs

50ml milk

1 tsp ground turmeric

5g parsley, finely chopped

Directions

In a skillet, heat the oil over high heat. Toss in the red onion and chili, frying for 2-3 minutes.

In a large bowl, whisk together the milk, parsley, eggs, and turmeric. Pour into the skillet and lower to medium heat. Cook for 3 to 5 minutes, scrambling the mixture as you do with a spoon or spatula. Serve immediately.

Nutrition:

Calories 113

Preparation Time: 10 minutes

Cooking Time: 20 minutes

Servings: 1

Ingredients

1 tsp tomato puree

1 star anise, squashed

Parsley

Coriander

Juice of ½ lime

500ml chicken stock

½ carrot, stripped and cut into matchsticks

50g broccoli, cut into little florets

50g beansprouts

100g raw tiger prawns

100g firm tofu

50g rice noodles, cooked by parcel

Directions

50g cooked water chestnuts

20g sushi ginger, sliced

1 tbsp great quality miso glue

Directions

Place the tomato puree, star anise, parsley stalks, coriander stalks, lime juice, and chicken stock in a huge container and bring to a stew for 10 minutes.

Include the carrot, broccoli, prawns, tofu, noodles, and water chestnuts and stew tenderly until the prawns are cooked through. Expel from the heat and mix in the sushi ginger and miso glue.

Serve sprinkled with the parsley and coriander leaves.

Nutrition:

Calories 345

Preparation Time: 10 minutes

Cooking Time: 25 minutes

Servings: 2

Ingredients

150g of turkey

150g of cauliflower

40g of red onion

1 teaspoon fresh ginger

1 bird's eye pepper

1 clove of garlic

3 tablespoons of extra virgin olive oil

2 teaspoons of turmeric

30g of dried tomatoes

10g of parsley

dried sage to taste

1 tablespoon of capers

1/4 of fresh lemon juice

Directions:

Blend the raw cauliflower tops and cook them in a teaspoon of extra virgin olive oil, garlic, red onion, chili pepper, ginger, and a teaspoon of turmeric. Leave to flavor for a minute, then add the chopped sun-dried tomatoes and 5g of parsley over the heat. Season the turkey slice with a teaspoon of extra virgin olive oil, the dried sage, and cook it in another teaspoon of extra virgin olive oil. Once ready, season with a tablespoon of capers, 1/4 of lemon juice, 5g of parsley, a tablespoon of water and add the cauliflower.

Nutrition:

Calories 482

80. Sirtfood Cocktail

Preparation Time: 10 minutes

Cooking Time: 0 minutes

Servings: 1

Ingredients

75g (3oz) kale

50g (2oz) strawberries

1 apple, cored

2 sticks of celery

1 tablespoon parsley

1 teaspoon of matcha powder

Squeeze lemon juice (optional) to taste

Nutrition:

Calories 122

Direction

Place the ingredients into a blender and add enough water to cover the ingredients and blitz to a smooth consistency.

Preparation Time: 10 minutes

Cooking Time: 0 minutes

Servings: 1

Ingredients

50g (2oz) blueberries

50g (2oz) strawberries

25g (1oz) blackcurrants

25g (1oz) red grapes

1 carrot, peeled

1 orange, peeled

Juice of 1 lime

Nutrition:

Calories 99

Direction

Place all of the ingredients into a blender and cover them with water. Blitz until smooth. You can also add some crushed ice and a mint leaf to garnish.

Preparation Time: 10 minutes

Cooking Time: 0 minutes

Servings: 1

Ingredients

1 stalk of celery

50g (2oz) kale

1 apple, cored

50g (2oz) mango, peeled, de-stoned and chopped

2.5cm (1 inch) chunk of fresh ginger root, peeled and chopped

Nutrition:

Calories 114

Direction

Put all the ingredients into a blender with some water and blitz until smooth. Add ice to make your smoothie really refreshing.

Preparation Time: 10 minutes

Cooking Time: 0 minutes

Servings: 1

Ingredients

1 carrot, peeled

1 orange, peeled

1 stick of celery

1 apple, cored

50g (2oz) kale

½ teaspoon matcha powder

Nutrition:

Calories 104

Direction

Place all of the ingredients into a blender and add in enough water to cover them. Process until smooth, serve, and enjoy.

Preparation Time: 10 minutes

Cooking Time: 0 minutes

Servings: 1

Ingredients

100g (3½ oz) strawberries

75g (3oz) frozen pitted cherries

1 tablespoon plain full-fat yogurt

175mls (6fl oz) unsweetened soya milk

.

Nutrition:

Calories 98

Direction

Place all of the ingredients into a blender and process until smooth. Serve and enjoy

Preparation Time: 10 minutes

Cooking Time: 0 minutes

Servings: 1

Ingredients

75g (3oz) red grapes

3 sticks of celery

1 avocado, de-stoned and peeled

1 tablespoon fresh parsley

½ teaspoon matcha powder

Nutrition:

Calories 113

Direction

Place all of the ingredients into a blender with enough water to cover them and blitz until smooth and creamy. Add crushed ice to make it even more refreshing.

Preparation Time: 10 minutes

Cooking Time: 0 minutes

Servings: 1

Ingredients

75g (3oz) strawberries

1 apple, cored

1 orange, peeled

½ avocado, peeled and de-stoned

½ teaspoon matcha powder

Juice of 1 lime

Direction

Place all of the ingredients into a blender with enough water to cover them and process until smooth.

Nutrition:

Calories 104

Preparation Time: 10 minutes

Cooking Time: 0 minutes

Servings: 1

Ingredients

1 grapefruit, peeled

2 stalks of celery

50g (2oz) kale

½ teaspoon matcha powder

Nutrition:

Calories 120

Direction

Place all the ingredients into a blender with enough water to cover them and blitz until smooth.

Preparation Time: 10 minutes

Cooking Time: 0 minutes

Servings: 1

Ingredients

1 carrot, peeled

3 stalks of celery

1 orange, peeled

½ teaspoon matcha powder

Juice of 1 lime

Nutrition:

Calories 117

Direction

Place all of the ingredients into a blender with enough water to cover them and blitz until smooth.

Preparation Time: 10 minutes

Cooking Time: 0 minutes

Servings: 1

Ingredients

1 mango, peeled & de-stoned

75g (3oz) fresh pineapple, chopped

50g (2oz) kale

25g (1oz) rocket

1 tablespoon 100% cocoa powder or cacao nibs

150mls (5fl oz) coconut milk

Nutrition:

Calories 121

Direction

Place all of the ingredients into a blender and blitz until smooth. You can add a little water if it seems too thick.

Bonus Recipes

90. Buckwheat Porridge

Preparation time: 10 minutes

Cooking time: 15 minutes

Servings: 2

Ingredients

1 cup buckwheat, rinsed

1 cup unsweetened almond milk

1 cup of water

½ teaspoon ground cinnamon

½ teaspoon vanilla extract

1–2 tablespoons raw honey

¼ cup fresh blueberries

Directions:

In a pan, add all the ingredients (except honey and blueberries) over medium-high heat and bring to a boil. Now, reduce the heat to low and simmer, covered for about 10 minutes. Stir in the honey and remove from the heat. Set aside, covered, for about 5 minutes. With a fork, fluff the mixture, and transfer into serving bowls. Top with blueberries and serve.

Nutrition:

Calories 358

Total Fat 4.7

Carbs 3.7 g

Sodium 95 m

Fiber 9.8 g

Protein 12 g

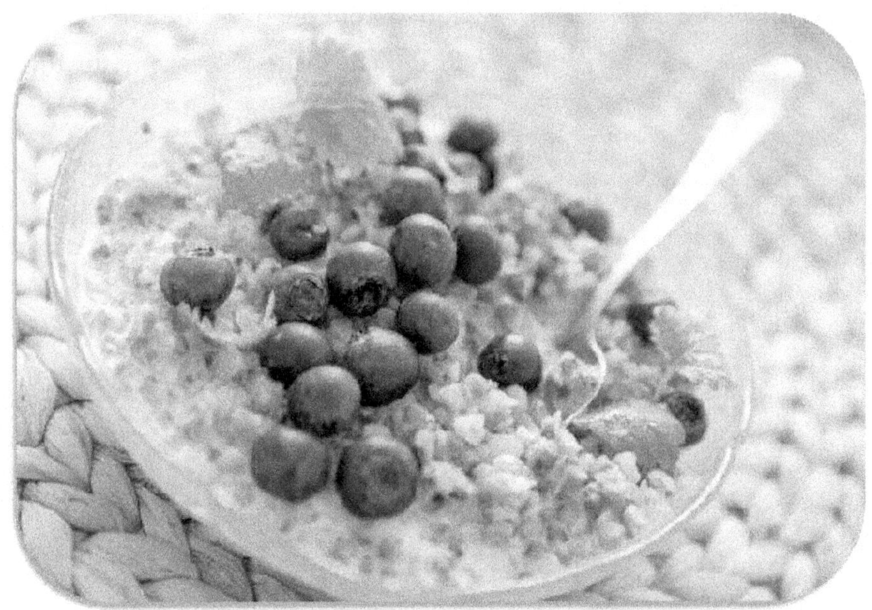

Preparation time: 10 minutes

Cooking time: 38 minutes

Servings: 8

Ingredients

¼ cup cacao powder

¼ cup maple syrup

2 tablespoons coconut oil, melted

½ teaspoon vanilla extract

1/8 teaspoon salt

2 cups gluten-free rolled oats

¼ cup unsweetened coconut flakes

2 tablespoons chia seeds

2 tablespoons unsweetened dark chocolate, chopped finely

Directions

Preheat your oven to 300°F and line a medium baking sheet with parchment paper. In a medium pan, add the cacao powder, maple syrup, coconut oil, vanilla extract, and salt, and mix well. Now, place the pan over medium heat and cook for about 2–3 minutes, or until thick and syrupy, stirring continuously. Remove from the heat and set aside. In a large bowl, add the oats, coconut, and chia seeds and mix well. Add the syrup mixture and mix until well combined. Transfer the granola mixture onto a prepared baking sheet and spread in an even layer. Bake for about 35 minutes. Remove from the oven and set aside for about 1 hour. Add the chocolate pieces and stir to combine. Serve immediately.

Nutritional Values

Calories 193

Total Fat 9.1 g

Carbs 26.1 g

Sodium 37 mg

Fiber 4.6 g

Protein 5 g

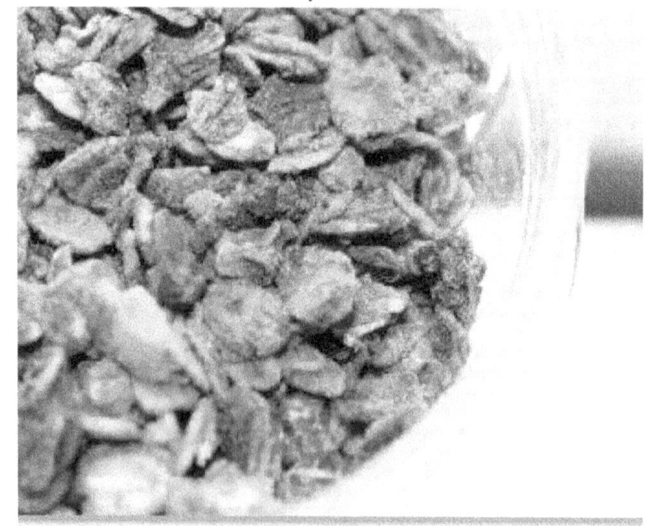

Preparation time: 15 minutes

Cooking time: 20 minutes

Servings: 8

Ingredients

1 cup buckwheat flour

¼ cup arrowroot starch

1½ teaspoons baking powder

¼ teaspoon of sea salt

2 eggs

½ cup unsweetened almond milk

2–3 tablespoons maple syrup

2 tablespoons coconut oil, melted

1 cup fresh blueberries

Directions:

Preheat your oven to 350°F and line 8 cups of a muffin tin. In a bowl, place the buckwheat flour, arrowroot starch, baking powder, and salt, and mix well. In a separate bowl, place the eggs, almond milk, maple syrup, and coconut oil, and beat until well combined. Now, place the flour mixture and mix until just combined. Gently, fold in the blueberries. Transfer the mixture into prepared muffin cups evenly. Bake for about 25 minutes or until a toothpick inserted in the center comes out clean. Remove the muffin tin from the oven and place onto a wire rack to cool for about 10 minutes. Carefully invert the muffins onto the wire rack to cool completely before serving.

Nutrition

Calories 136

Total Fat 5.3 g

Saturated Fat 3.4 g

Cholesterol 41 mg

Sodium 88 mg

Total Carbs 20.7 g

Fiber 2.2 g

Sugar 5.7 g

Protein 3.5 g

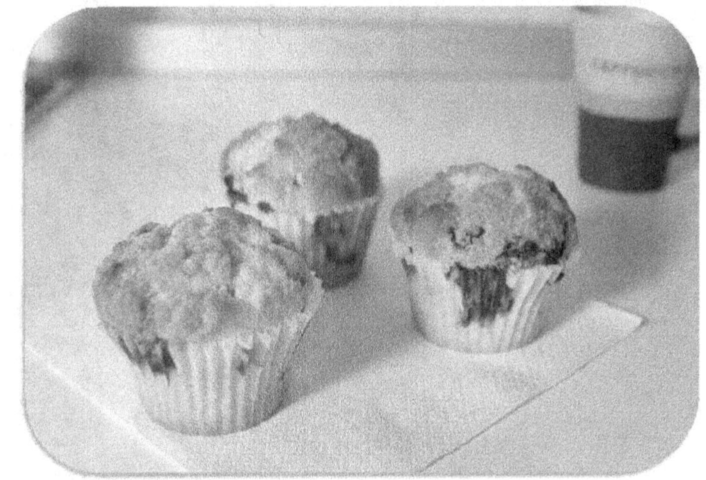

Preparation time: 15 minutes

Cooking time: 24 minutes

Servings: 8

Ingredients

2 cups unsweetened almond milk

1 tablespoon fresh lemon juice

1 cup buckwheat flour

½ cup cacao powder

¼ cup flaxseed meal

1 teaspoon baking soda

1 teaspoon baking powder

¼ teaspoons kosher salt

2 large eggs

½ cup coconut oil, melted

¼ cup dark brown sugar

2 teaspoons vanilla extract

2 ounces unsweetened dark chocolate, chopped roughly

Nutrition:

Calories 295

Total Fat 22.1 g

Carbs 1.5 g

Sodium 302 mg

Fiber 5.2 g

Protein 6.3 g

Directions:

In a bowl, add the almond milk and lemon juice and mix well. Set aside for about 10 minutes. In a bowl, place buckwheat flour, cacao powder, flaxseed meal, baking soda, baking powder, and salt, and mix well. In the bowl of the almond milk mixture, place the eggs, coconut oil, brown sugar, and vanilla extract and beat until smooth. Now, place the flour mixture and beat until smooth. Gently fold in the chocolate pieces. Preheat the waffle iron and then grease it. Place the desired amount of the mixture into the preheated waffle iron and cook for about 3 minutes, or until golden brown. Repeat with the remaining mixture.

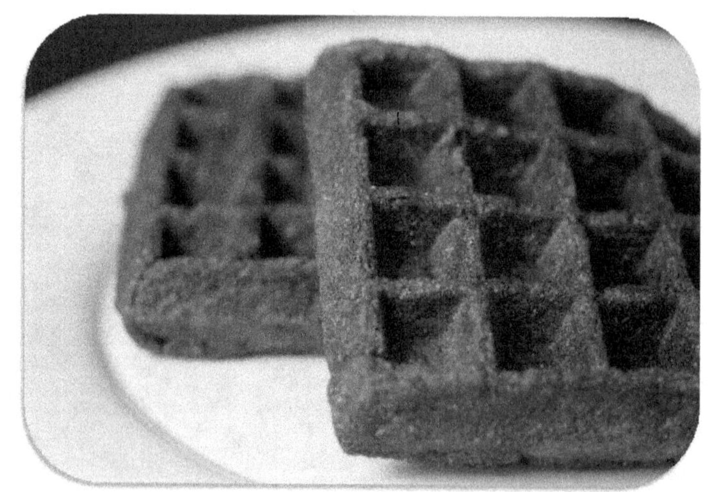

Preparation time: 10 minutes

Cooking time: 7 minutes

Servings: 4

Ingredients

6 eggs

2 tablespoons unsweetened almond milk

Salt and ground black pepper, to taste

2 tablespoons olive oil

4 ounces smoked salmon, cut into bite-sized chunks

2 cup fresh kale, tough ribs removed and chopped finely

4 scallions, chopped finely

Directions:

In a bowl, place the eggs, coconut milk, salt, and black pepper and beat well. Set aside. In a non-stick wok, heat the oil over medium heat. Place the egg mixture evenly and cook for about 30 seconds without stirring. Place the salmon kale and scallions on top of the egg mixture evenly. Now, reduce heat to low. With the lid, cover the wok and cook for about 4–5 minutes or until the omelet is done completely. Uncover the wok and cook for about 1 minute. Carefully transfer the omelet onto a serving plate and serve.

Nutritional Values

Calories 210

Total Fat 14.9 g

Sodium 682 mg

Carbs 5.2 g

Fiber 0.9 g

Protein 14.8 g

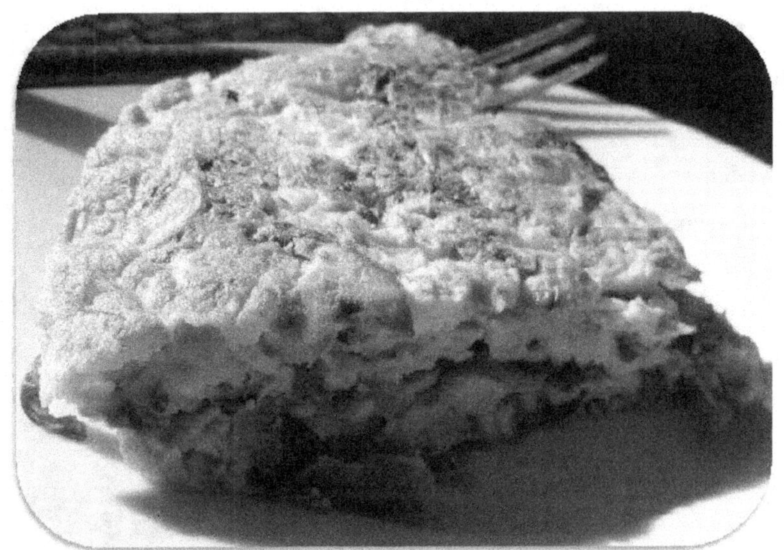

95. Eggs with Kale

Preparation time: 15 minutes

Cooking time: 25 minutes

Servings: 4

Ingredients

2 tablespoons olive oil

1 yellow onion, chopped

2 garlic cloves, minced

1 cup tomatoes, chopped

½ pound fresh kale, tough ribs removed and chopped

1 teaspoon ground cumin

¼ teaspoon red pepper flakes, crushed

Salt and ground black pepper, to taste

4 eggs

2 tablespoons fresh parsley, chopped

Directions:

Heat the oil in a large wok over medium heat and sauté the onion for about 4–5 minutes. Add garlic and sauté for about 1 minute. Add the tomatoes, spices, salt, and black pepper and cook for about 2–3 minutes, stirring frequently. Stir in the kale and cook for about 4–5 minutes. Carefully, crack eggs on top of the kale mixture. With the lid, cover the wok and cook for about 10 minutes, or until the desired doneness of eggs. Serve hot with the garnishing of parsley.

Nutritional Values

Calories 175

Fat 11.7 g

Carbs 11.5 g

Sodium 130 mg

Fiber 2.2 g

Protein 8.2 g

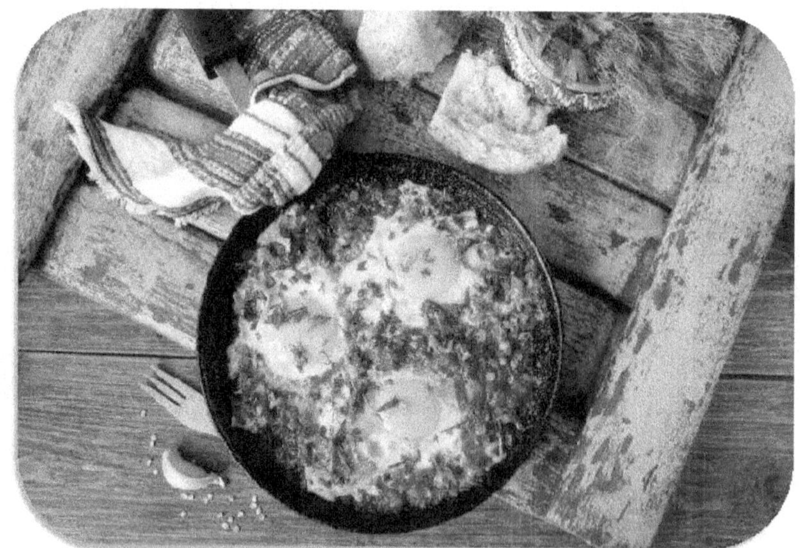

Exercising

Combining Exercise with the Sirtfood Diet

With 52% of Americans admitting that they discover it simpler to do their taxes than to comprehend how to consume healthily, it's crucial to introduce a kind of eating that becomes a lifestyle rather than a one-off crash diet. For a few of us, it may not be that tough to drop weight or retain a healthy weight; however, the Sirtfood diet plan can assist those who are struggling. What about integrating the Sirtfood diet plan with a workout, is it a good idea to prevent exercise entirely or present it when you have begun the diet plan?

The SirtDiet Principles

With an estimated 650 million obese adults globally, it's essential to find healthy eating and exercise routines that are achievable, don't deny you of whatever you delight in, and don't require you to work out all week. The bright side is that particular food and beverage, consisting of dark chocolate and red wine, consists of chemicals called polyphenols that trigger the genes that imitate the results of exercise and fasting.

Exercise During The First Few Weeks

During the very first week or two of the diet plan where your calories intake is minimized, it would be sensible to stop or lower workout while your body will adapt for fewer calories. Listen to your body, and don't force yourself if you feel like you are too tired, then don't exercise. Rather ensure that you stay focused on the principles that use to a healthy lifestyle such as consisting of sufficient everyday levels of fiber, protein and fruit, and veggies.

When The Diet Becomes A Lifestyle

If you are doing your exercise, it's important to take in protein, preferably an hour after your workout. Protein repair work muscles after a workout, lowers pain, and can aid healing. The kind of physical fitness you do will be down to you; however, exercises in the house will permit you to select when to exercise, the types of workouts that fit you and are short and hassle-free.

The Sirtfood diet is a fantastic way to change your eating practices, reduce weight, and feel healthier. The preliminary few weeks may challenge you, but it is necessary to examine which foods are best to consume and which scrumptious recipes match you. Be kind to your body in the first couple of weeks. If you are already somebody who does extreme or moderate exercise, then it might be that you can continue as typical or manage your physical fitness in accordance with the change in diet. Similar to any diet plan and workout changes, it's everything about the private and how far you can press yourself.

Home body weight circuit training:

- 30 seconds of bodyweight squats, or until you can't do anymore (might be less than 30 seconds in the beginning)
- 30 seconds of push-ups, or until you can't do anymore (might be less than 30 seconds in the beginning)
- 30 seconds jumping jacks

Repeat 3-4 times.

This is very basic training that will lead you into strength type exercising. When you can do this easily every morning (or every second morning), you can add into every circuit following:

- 20 walking lunges
- 15-30 seconds plank

And even more advanced body weight circuit training would be to add pull ups, dips (using bar stools) and chin ups and repeat whole circuit for 5 times. That should have sweat you like a pig and your metabolism should be running full steam. So, advanced body circuit training might be:

- 20 bodyweight squats

You may repeat the two phases as often as you would like to meet your weight loss goals. Even if you have achieved it, the creators of the diet suggest adopting sirtfoods for your day-to-day needs because they have designed this diet as an alternative way of living.

This means that after the first three weeks, you are encouraged to keep having meals and green juices that are rich in sirtfoods. Other than this, here are some more things that you can do to get more and continue reaping the benefits of sirtfoods for your health:

Resume Your Workout Routines.

Since your calorie limit for the first couple of weeks into the diet, it is best to either lessen or stop working out while your body gets used to its new condition. No two persons are exactly alike, so the best thing you can do to know when you can start exercising like you usually do it by paying closer attention to your body.

To be on the safer side of things, most followers opt to resume their regular workout schedule after clearing phase 2 of the diet. By then, you would feel more energized, and more capable of completing your usual exercise sets.

Take note that even though a sirtfood diet does not require you to exercise to unlock its benefits, it would still be best for the overall wellness of your body and mind to remain fit and active every day.

Try Out Sirtfood Smoothies With Protein Powder.

If you decide to start exercising again, you should add smoothies that contain lots of sirtfoods and protein powder to help you reduce the soreness of your muscles, and keep you well energized throughout and after your workout.

Recipes for fun and tasty sirtfood smoothies can easily be found in blogs and recipe books dedicated to the Sirtfood Diet. If you are pretty confident with your skills in the kitchen, then feel free to experiment with the recommended ingredients, and discover the perfect smoothie combinations for your taste buds.

Invite your family and friends to try out the diet.

One of the best ways to maintain your healthier diet is by getting the people around you involved in it as well. Studies show that the kind of company you keep can have a huge influence on your lifestyle, including what and how you eat.

Ideally, you can try convincing them by showing the positive effects that the Sirtfood Diet has had on you. Let them also read this guide so that they will have a better idea of what it is, what it can do for them, and how they should go about it.

Consider adopting the principles of the Sirtfood Diet as part of your way of life. It is just not a one-time, quick-fix meal plan, and you cannot go wrong by adding more sirtfoods into your day-to-day diet.

Is It Healthy And Sustainable?

Sirtfoods are nearly all healthy options and may even lead to some health benefits due to their anti-inflammatory or antioxidant residential or commercial properties.

The Sirtfood Diet is needlessly restrictive and uses no clear, special health benefits over any other kind of diet.

Eating only 1,000 calories is normally not suggested without the supervision of a physician. Even consuming 1,500 calories per day is exceedingly limiting for many individuals.

The diet plan also needs draining to 3 green juices per day. Although juices can be a good source of minerals and vitamins, they are likewise a source of sugar and consist of nearly none of the healthy fiber that whole fruits and veggies do

What's more, sipping on juice throughout the whole day is a bad concept for both your blood sugar and your teeth.

Conclusion

Traditional diets are based on decreasing calories, a very effective approach for those who want to lose excess weight. On the other hand, however, there is an increase in the desire for prohibited foods from a psychological point of view, with binge eating that risks frustrating the work done with the diet. To avoid this frustration, Sirt Diet intervenes to help, because it is based on the inclusion and not on the exclusion of food, without particular renunciations.

The Latin motto "mens sana in corpore sano" represents a valid expression of that healthy ambition that each individual should cultivate. The incorrect intake of food can be one of the main factors in the onset of diseases due to an excess of introduced calories, compared to those consumed. If sedentary lifestyles are added to this, the risk of incurring overweight and obesity becomes a certainty. The low-calories Sirt diet is essentially based on a reasoned and varied combination of foods, and a diet aimed at achieving weight loss with the harmonious development of the organism.

For this reason, it is necessary to replace a traditional low-calories food program with all that sirtfoods offer. The purpose of this diet is to accompany and support the individual during a not simple process of change, which involves the acquisition of a different dietary and physical lifestyle.

Avoiding many tasty foods is a bad habit because the body is deprived of the necessary need for important nutrients. The lean genes responsible for repairing and rejuvenating cells accelerate their activity by drawing on fat reserves and increasing disease resistance. The same goal can be achieved without starving, by eating genetically rich Sirtfoods, "sirtuins," considered to be super regulators of metabolism. They influence our ability to burn fat, the mechanisms that regulate longevity, mood, and improve memory.

A complete approach to embarking on a new lifestyle is achieved when the diet is integrated with physical activity. Healthy eating behavior places the person's wellness philosophy at the center of attention, to foster a state of psychophysical balance. Achieving a correct bodyweight must be achieved both by controlling nutrition and by making a more physically active life. Only in this way it is possible to prevent obesity and other pathologies.

Considering that to this must be added environmental and genetic risk factors, the complexity of the elements involved makes it clear that it is necessary to intervene, where possible, in an early manner.

In particular, as regards nutrition, prevention on eating must start from childhood and should become a heritage for the personal culture of every human being.

In many countries, with the aim of providing indications on how to eat, public institutions and scientific bodies have developed specific guidelines, aimed at defining and disseminating the basic information for a balanced diet aimed at well-being.

www.ingramcontent.com/pod-product-compliance
Lightning Source LLC
Chambersburg PA
CBHW081231250726
48654CB00012B/1294